More Case Studies in Stroke

Common and Uncommon Presentations

More Case Studies in Stroke

Common and Uncommon Presentations

Edited by

Michael G. Hennerici

Professor of Neurology,
Chairman at the Department of Neurology,
UniversitätsMedizin Mannheim,
University of Heidelberg, Mannheim, Germany

Rolf Kern

Professor of Neurology at the Department of Neurology,
UniversitätsMedizin Mannheim,
University of Heidelberg, Mannheim, Germany

Louis R. Caplan

Professor of Neurology, Senior Neurologist,
Beth Israel Deaconess Medical Center,
Harvard Medical School, Boston, MA, USA

Kristina Szabo

Professor of Neurology at the Department of Neurology,
UniversitätsMedizin Mannheim,
University of Heidelberg, Mannheim, Germany

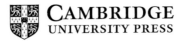

CAMBRIDGE
UNIVERSITY PRESS

CAMBRIDGE
UNIVERSITY PRESS

University Printing House, Cambridge CB2 8BS, United Kingdom

Cambridge University Press is part of the University of Cambridge.

It furthers the University's mission by disseminating knowledge in the pursuit of
education, learning and research at the highest international levels of excellence.

www.cambridge.org
Information on this title: www.cambridge.org/9781107610033

© Cambridge University Press 2014

First published 2014

Printed in Spain by Grafos SA, Arte sobre papel

A catalogue record for this publication is available from the British Library

Library of Congress Cataloguing in Publication data
More case studies in stroke : common and uncommon presentations / [edited by] Michael G. Hennerici,
Rolf Kern, Louis R. Caplan, Kristina Szabo.
       p.   cm.
Preceded by: Case studies in stroke / edited by Michael G. Hennerici, et al. 2007.
Includes bibliographical references.
ISBN 978-1-107-61003-3 (Paperback)
I.   Hennerici, M. (Michael), editor of compilation.   II.   Kern, Rolf, editor of compilation.   III.   Caplan,
Louis R., editor of compilation.   IV.   Szabo, Kristina, editor of compilation.   V.   Case studies in stroke.
Preceded by (work): [DNLM: 1.   Stroke–diagnosis–Case Reports.   2.   Diagnostic Techniques, Neurological–
Case Reports.   3.   Neurologic Manifestations–Case Reports.   4.   Stroke–therapy–Case Reports. WL 356]
RC388.5
616.8′1–dc23   2013041805

ISBN 978-1-107-61003-3 Paperback

Contents

Section 3. Stroke mimics

The following cases described herein have been published previously:

Case 8.   Bolognese M, Griebe M, Foerster A, Hennerici MG, Fatar M. Thrombolytic stroke treatment of a 12-year-old girl with intracranial fibromuscular dysplasia. *Case Rep Neurol* 2011; **3**(3): 210–13.

Case 12.   Menzel T, Kern R, Griebe M, Hennerici M, Fatar M. Acute posterior ischemic optic neuropathy mimicking posterior cerebral artery stroke visualized by 3-tesla MRI. *Case Rep Neurol* 2012; **4**(3): 173–6.

Case 35.   Szabo K, Achtnichts L, Grips E, et al. Stroke-like presentation in a case of Creutzfeldt–Jakob disease. *Cerebrovasc Dis* 2004; **18**: 251–3.

Case 36.   Reuter B, Wolf ME, Förster A, et al. Stroke-like presentation of toxic leukoencephalopathy as the initial manifestation of HIV infection. *Case Rep Neurol* 2012; **4**(3): 231–5.

List of contributors

Sefanja Achterberg
Department of Neurology, Utrecht
Stroke Center, Rudolf Magnus Institute
of Neuroscience University Medical
Center Utrecht, Utrecht, the
Netherlands

James A. Adams
Royal Surrey County Hospital NHS
Foundation Trust, Surrey, UK

Angelika Alonso
Department of Neurology,
UniversitätsMedizin Mannheim,
University of Heidelberg, Mannheim,
Germany

Bettina Anders
Department of Neurology,
UniversitätsMedizin Mannheim,
University of Heidelberg, Mannheim,
Germany

Ana Patrícia Antunes
Neurology Department, Hospital Santa
Maria, Lisbon, Portugal

Johannes Binder
Zentrum für Nervenheilkunde
Herbolzheim, Herbolzheim,
Germany

Manuel Bolognese
Department of Neurology,
UniversitätsMedizin Mannheim,
University of Heidelberg, Mannheim,
Germany

Louis R. Caplan
Beth Israel Deaconess Medical Center,
Division of Cerebrovascular Stroke,
Boston, MA, USA

Paolo Costa
Department of Clinical Neurology,
University of Brescia, Italy

Sofie De Blauwe
Department of Neurology, Antwerp
University Hospital, Antwerp, the
Netherlands

Exuperio Díez-Tejedor
Department of Neurology and Stroke
Centre, La Paz University Hospital,
Autónoma of Madrid University;
Neurosciences Area of IdiPAZ Health
Research Institute, Madrid, Spain

Philipp Eisele
Department of Neurology,
UniversitätsMedizin Mannheim,
University of Heidelberg, Mannheim,
Germany

Alex Förster
Department of Neurology,
UniversitätsMedizin Mannheim,
University of Heidelberg, Mannheim,
Germany

Blanca Fuentes
Department of Neurology and Stroke
Centre, La Paz University Hospital,
Autónoma of Madrid University;
Neurosciences Area of IdiPAZ Health
Research Institute, Madrid, Spain

Ruth Geraldes
Neurology Department, Hospital Santa
Maria, Lisbon, Portugal

Martin Griebe
Department of Neurology,
UniversitätsMedizin Mannheim,
University of Heidelberg, Mannheim,
Germany

Valentin Held
Department of Neurology,
UniversitätsMedizin Mannheim,
University of Heidelberg, Mannheim,
Germany

Gregory Helsen
Department of Neurology,
General Hospital St. Elisabeth,
Herentals,
Belgium

Michael G. Hennerici
Department of Neurology,
UniversitätsMedizin Mannheim,
University of Heidelberg, Mannheim,
Germany

Eva Hornberger
Department of Neurology,
UniversitätsMedizin Mannheim,
University of Heidelberg, Mannheim,
Germany

Micha Kablau
Department of Neurology,
UniversitätsMedizin Mannheim,
University of Heidelberg, Mannheim,
Germany

L. Jaap Kappelle
Department of Neurology, Utrecht
Stroke Center, Rudolf Magnus Institute
of Neuroscience University Medical
Center Utrecht, Utrecht, the Netherlands

Rolf Kern
Department of Neurology,
UniversitätsMedizin Mannheim,
University of Heidelberg, Mannheim,
Germany

Patricia Martínez-Sánchez
Department of Neurology and Stroke
Centre, La Paz University Hospital,
Autónoma of Madrid University;
Neurosciences Area of IdiPAZ Health
Research Institute, Madrid, Spain

Tilman Menzel
Department of Neurology,
UniversitätsMedizin Mannheim,
University of Heidelberg, Mannheim,
Germany

Nadja Meyer
Department of Neurology,
UniversitätsMedizin Mannheim,

University of Heidelberg, Mannheim,
Germany

Caroline Ottomeyer
Department of Neurology,
UniversitätsMedizin Mannheim,
University of Heidelberg, Mannheim,
Germany

Suzanne Persoon
Department of Neurology, Utrecht
Stroke Center, Rudolf Magnus Institute
of Neuroscience University Medical
Center Utrecht, Utrecht, the
Netherlands

Alessandro Pezzini
Department of Clinical Neurology,
University of Brescia, Italy

Miriam M. Pfeiffer
Department of Neurology,
Katholisches Klinikum Koblenz,
Koblenz, Germany

Björn Reuter
Department of Neurology,
UniversitätsMedizin Mannheim,
University of Heidelberg, Mannheim,
Germany

Katlijn Schotsmans
Department of Neurology, Antwerp
University Hospital, Antwerp, the
Netherlands

Christopher Schwarzbach
Department of Neurology,
UniversitätsMedizin Mannheim,
University of Heidelberg, Mannheim,
Germany

Markus Stürmlinger
Department of Neurology,
UniversitätsMedizin Mannheim,
University of Heidelberg, Mannheim,
Germany

Kristina Szabo
Department of Neurology,
UniversitätsMedizin Mannheim,
University of Heidelberg, Mannheim,
Germany

Tiago Teodoro
Neurology Department, Hospital Santa
Maria, Lisbon, Portugal

Ralph Werner
Department of Neurology, Katholisches
Klinikum Koblenz, Koblenz, Germany

Johannes C. Wöhrle
Department of Neurology,
Katholisches Klinikum Koblenz,
Koblenz, Germany

Marc Wolf
Department of Neurology,
UniversitätsMedizin Mannheim,
University of Heidelberg, Mannheim,
Germany

Preface

In 1851, the French physician Paul Pierre Broca presented the brain of a patient named Leborgne, who during his lifetime had suffered from a loss of speech with preserved comprehension and had died at the age of 51 due to an infected gangrene. At autopsy, Broca found destruction of the dorsal part of the left inferior frontal gyrus. Broca termed the loss of articulated speech *aphémie;* today, expressive aphasia is also known as Broca's aphasia. The case of the patient Leborgne is not only one of the most famous case reports in neurology, it is also an excellent example of how instructive such individual cases can be for today's neurologists – even historical ones. Case number 14 in this book describes a stroke patient who presented with aphemia, a rare and isolated disorder of the planning of motor articulation of speech. During his hospital stay, we reverted to Broca's case several times to understand the syndrome of our patient better. In addition to basic stroke research and large randomized clinical trials to establish recommendations for prevention and management of acute cerebrovascular events, individual case reports reflecting the day-to-day experience of academic physicians open a wealth of fascinating perspectives for future research.

The second volume of *Case Studies in Stroke - Common and Uncommon Presentations* is a collection of 42 in-depth case studies, partly from our department in Mannheim but also from presenters at the European Stroke Conference 2011 in Hamburg, and from participants of the 15th ESO Stroke Summer School, which took place in Mannheim and Heidelberg in July 2011. We are very grateful to Louis Caplan–one of the pioneers of stroke research with exceptional clinical experience–for not only contributing his own cases but also reading and discussing all presentations with us. We hope that the readers will enjoy the book as much as we did preparing it and that the lessons learned will assist them in providing better care for their patients.

Michael G. Hennerici
Rolf Kern
Louis R. Caplan
Kristina Szabo

Abbreviations

ACA	anterior cerebral artery
ACE	angiotensin-converting enzyme
ADC	apparent diffusion coefficient (MRI)
aPTT	activated partial thromboplastin time
ASCO	atherosclerosis–small vessel disease–cardiac source–other (score)
ASD	atrial septal defect
AVM	arteriovenous malformation
CAA	cerebral amyloid angiopathy
CEA	carotid endarterectomy
CNS	central nervous system
CRP	C-reactive protein
CSF	cerebrospinal fluid
CT	computed tomography
CTA	computed tomography angiography
CVT	cerebral venous thrombosis
DVT	deep vein thrombosis
DWI	diffusion-weighted imaging (MRI)
ECASS	European Cooperative Acute Stroke Study
ECG	electrocardiogram
EEG	electroencephalography
EP	evoked potential
EVD	external ventricular drain
FLAIR	fluid-attenuated inversion recovery (MRI)
fMRI	functional MRI
GCS	Glasgow Coma Scale
GFAP	glial fibrillary acidic protein
HaNDL	headache with neurological deficits and CSF lymphocytosis
HITS	high-intensity transient signals (Doppler sonography)
IAT	intra-arterial thrombolysis
ICA	internal carotid artery
ICH	intracerebral hemorrhage
ICU	intensive care unit

INR	international normalized ratio
IVT	intravenous thrombolysis
LMWH	low molecular weight heparin
MCA	middle cerebral artery
MELAS	mitochondrial encephalomyopathy, lactic acidosis, and stroke-like episodes
MMSE	mini-mental state examination
MRA	magnetic resonance angiography
MRI	magnetic resonance imaging
mRS	modified Rankin Scale
NBTE	non-bacterial thrombotic endocarditis
NIHSS	National Institutes of Health Stroke Scale
NINDS	National Institute of Neurological Disorders and Stroke
NSAIDs	nonsteroidal anti-inflammatory drugs
OHSS	ovarian hyperstimulation syndrome
PCA	posterior cerebral artery
PCI	percutaneous coronary intervention
PCR	polymerase chain reaction
PET	positron emission tomography
PFO	patent foramen ovale
PIB	Pittsburgh compound-B
PICA	posterior inferior cerebellar artery
PION	posterior ischemic optic neuropathy
PRES	posterior reversible encephalopathy syndrome
PWI	perfusion-weighted imaging (MRI)
RCTs	randomized clinical trials
r-tPA	recombinant tissue plasminogen activator
SAH	subarachnoid hemorrhage
sCAD	spontaneous cervical artery dissection
SSRI	serotonin-specific reuptake inhibitors
SVE	subcortical vascular encephalopathy
TAAD	thoracic aortic aneurysms and dissections
TCCS	transcranial color-coded duplex sonography
TCD	transcranial Doppler sonography
TEE	transesophageal echocardiography
TIA	transient ischemic attack
TOF	time-of-flight
tPA	tissue plasminogen activator
TTE	transthoracic echocardiography
VA	vertebral artery
VAD	vertebral artery dissection

Introduction: approach to the patient

It happened on April 13, 1737, as "the whole house vibrated from a dull thud...something huge and heavy must have crashed down on the upper floor." The servant of the composer George Frederick Handel ran up the stairs to his master's workroom and found him "lying lifeless on the floor, eyes staring open..." Handel had come home from the rehearsal in a furious rage, his face bright red, his temples pulsating. He had slammed the house door and then stamped about, as the servant could hear, on the first floor back and forth so that the ceiling rebounded: it wasn't advisable, on such anger-filled days, to be casual in your service.

From the lower floor Christopher Smith, the master's assistant, went upstairs; he had also been shocked by the thud. He ran to fetch the doctor for the royal composer. "How old is he?" "Fifty-two," answered Smith. "Terrible age, he had worked like an ox." Dr. Jenkins bent deeply over him. "He is, however, strong as an ox. Now we will see what he can do." He noticed that one eye, the right one, stared lifeless and the other one reacted. He tried to lift the right arm. It fell back lifeless. He then lifted the left one. The left one stayed in the new position. Now Dr. Jenkins knew enough. As he left the room, Smith followed him to the stairs, worried. "What is it?" "Apoplexia. The right side is paralysed." "And will..." Smith formed the words–"will he recover?" Dr. Jenkins laboriously took a pinch of snuff. He didn't like such questions. "Perhaps. Anything is possible."

This colorful excerpt from the famous story *George Frederick Handel's Resurrection* by Stefan Zweig illustrates a long-lasting dilemma for doctor and patient after an acute stroke: the question of diagnosis and prognosis.

Today, 260 years after George Frederick Handel's stroke, Dr. Jenkins' successors are informed better about the pathomechanisms involved in the acute situation; for example, ischemia versus hemorrhage, cardio- and arterioembolic versus hemodynamic sources of ischemia, or small-vessel versus large-vessel disease. Even less common etiologies can be identified by additional tests (e.g., cerebrospinal fluid [CSF], biomarker and antibody tests). The benefits of acute therapy with a view to the different etiologies have risen, and the prognosis can be estimated more accurately: small cerebral hemorrhages or lacunar ischemic lesions have a good prognosis, both

More Case Studies in Stroke, eds. Michael G. Hennerici, Rolf Kern, Louis R. Caplan, and Kristina Szabo. Published by Cambridge University Press. © Cambridge University Press 2014.

being related to chronic, often inadequately treated hypertension in patients with subcortical vascular encephalopathy (SVE); this was most likely the cause of Handel's stroke. In addition, we have begun to elucidate the mechanisms of recovery after stroke. Functional magnetic resonance imaging (fMRI) and studies with positron emission tomography (PET) have shown that, following ischemic damage to either cerebral hemisphere, residual connections to corresponding remote areas can be activated and that even new synapses and neural network transformations are possible. These new findings have updated previous misconceptions regarding lack of plasticity in the adult human brain. Many of these new techniques have limited the application of our nearly outdated traditional tests (e.g., conventional angiography).

Nevertheless, the clinical case still presents a challenge for our colleagues in medicine, whether they are students, residents, or physicians with advanced expertise in stroke care. Like Dr. Jenkins, generations of physicians and neurologists in particular have based their diagnosis on a combination of (a) temporal profiles of illnesses, and (b) the presence or absence of focal, common, or uncommon signs and symptoms of stroke to conclude on the likely pathogenesis and pathobiology. The editors and contributors of this new book have tried to extend the series of common and uncommon stroke cases published in 2007 and to discuss key elements, whether they are clinical, brain and vascular imaging derived, or of other types of individual workup. Beyond traditional concepts and performance, the actual principle "time is brain" or probably "penumbra is brain" for stroke patients is illustrated, and consequently, clinical evaluation as well as technological studies are speeded-up; rather than traditional neurological examin-ations, a short but sufficient and therapy-related diagnosis-restricted repertoire is essential and includes all aspects of respiratory and cardiovascular function, as well as scores of the level of consciousness (using the Glasgow Coma Scale [GCS]) (Figure 1) and neurological and behavioral deficits (using the National Institutes of Health Stroke Scale [NIHSS]) (Figure 2). Detailed investigation should be avoided, but medical and surgical history from patients and their relatives still are to be carefully considered with regard to previous stroke events, treatments for other cardiovascular diseases, etc.

Standard technical tests include:

(i) electrocardiogram (ECG),
(ii) chest X-ray,
(iii) blood sample studies/blood cell counts (including thrombocytes) glucose, creatinine, creatinine in kinase or troponin and HS-troponin, electrolytes, international normalized ratio (INR), activated partial thromboplastin time (aPTT), and toxic substance quinine.

An ECG should always be carried out because of the high incidence of heart conditions in this population. Stroke and myocardial infarction may occur together. Arrhythmias frequently are either the cause or the result of embolic stroke.

Glasgow Coma Scale

Best eye response	Eye opening spontaneously	4
	Eye opening on command	3
	Eye opening to pain	2
	No eye opening	1
Best verbal response	Oriented	5
	Confused	4
	Inappropriate words	3
	Incomprehensible words	2
	No verbal response	1
Best motor response	Obeys commands	6
	Purposeful movement to pain	5
	Withdraws from pain	4
	Abnormal flexion to pain	3
	Extension to pain	2
	No motor response	1

Figure 1.   Glasgow Coma Outcome Scale.

Echocardiography should be performed as well in most patients with stroke to document any cardioembolic source (thrombus in the left atrium or atrial septal aneurysm) or an atheroma in the arch of the aorta. Equally, an echocardiogram is necessary to detect a shunt of blood from the right to the left atrium through a patent foramen ovale (PFO) or atrial septal defect (ASD). The accuracy of this ultrasound examination is greatly increased by transesophageal echocardiography (TEE) and transcranial Doppler sonography (TCD) studies as well as vascular computed tomography (CT)/magnetic resonance imaging (MRI) of the aortic arch.

In the acute situation, a separation between transient ischemic attack (TIA) and stroke is impossible and this term should not be accepted any longer, not least as both prognosis and course of the disease are similar – acute cerebrovascular syndrome is an appropriate alternative.

The same diagnostic studies are used for all patients with brain attacks, whether ischemic or hemorrhagic events, are suspected: both groups need CT/MRI of the brain and vessels including full cardiological workup (Figures 3 and 4).

CT is the standard method in both the acute and follow-up evaluation of cerebrovascular diseases, since its introduction in the early 1970s. Advantages of MRI are: excellent tissue contrast, high sensitivity for detecting early ischemic findings including brainstem and cerebellum, and high susceptibility for

NIH Stroke Scale

Assess level of consciousness

Alert	0
Drowsy	1
Stuporous	2
Coma	3

Assess orientation (month, age)

Both correctly	0
One correctly	1
Two incorrect	2

Follow commands
(1. Open and close eyes
2. Make fist and release)

Obeys both correctly	0
Obeys one correctly	1
Two incorrect	2

Follow my finger

Normal	0
Partial gaze palsy	1
Forced deviation	2

Visual field

Normal	0
Partial hemianopia	1
Complete hemianopia	2
Bilateral loss	3

Facial palsy

(Show teeth, raise eyebrows, squeeze
eyes shut)

Normal	0
Minor paralysis	1
Partial paralysis	2
Complete paralysis	3

Motor strength for each of four limbs
(Passively move extremity and observe strength)
a. Elevate left arm to 90 degrees
b. Elevate right arm to 90 degrees
c. Elevate left leg to 30 degrees
d. Elevate right leg to 30 degrees

No drift	0
Drift	1
Some effort against gravity	2
No effort against gravity	3
No movement	4
Amputation, joint fusion (untestable)	9

Co-ordination of limb ataxia

Absent	0
Present in upper or lower	1
Present in both	2

Sensory
(1. Pin prick to face, arm, trunk, and legs
2. Compare sides)

Normal	0
Partial loss	1
Dense loss	2

Speech clarity while reading word list

Normal articulation	0
Mild-moderate slurring	1
Nearly unintelligible, mute	2
Intubated or other physical barrier	9

Language (Describe picture, name items,
read sentences)

No aphasia	0
Mild-moderate aphasia	1
Severe aphasia	2
Mute	3

Extinction and inattention

No neglect	0
Partial neglect	1
Profound neglect	2

Total

Figure 2.   National Institutes of Health Stroke Scale.

demonstration of even very small hemorrhagic findings. Detection of flow parameters are excellent, although delineation of acute and developing penumbra surrounding the ischemic core or infarction are still insufficient as are sometimes developing ischemic territories close to parenchymal hemorrhage. Already approved early, specific stroke treatment with tissue plasminogen activator (tPA) requires CT within a short time frame of 4.5 hours. Beyond this time limit,

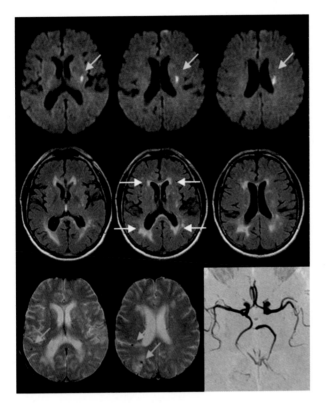

Figure 3.   Typical MRI findings in a 78-year-old stroke patient with cerebral microangiopathy. DWI (upper row) shows a single hyperintense acute ischemic lesion in the territory of a perforating artery (arrow). The T2-weighted FLAIR technique (middle row) demonstrates quite extensive chronic white matter lesions in a pattern typical for SVE with hyperintense lesions in the para- and periventricular white matter. T2* susceptibility-weighted sequences (bottom left and middle) show several small cortical/subcortical microbleeds, while the MRA (bottom right) demonstrates irregular contrast of intracranial vessels–a finding suggestive of arteriosclerosis.

successful treatment can be established only if MRI or specific CT methodologies are used, facilitating separation of perfusion deficits surrounding the core of already developing tissue necrosis (i.e., an equivalent of the ischemic penumbra) or if "bridging techniques" are used experimentally.

Conventional angiography, first performed in 1927, is selectively used only in very few acute stroke patients today for diagnostic purposes, but is still considered for early interventional treatment. Despite encouraging and evidence-based results of intra-arterial thrombolysis (IAT) in the carotid system and the basilar artery in randomized clinical trials (RCTs), current indications for angiography are left to patients with suspected vascular malformations or bleeding aneurysms. They

A

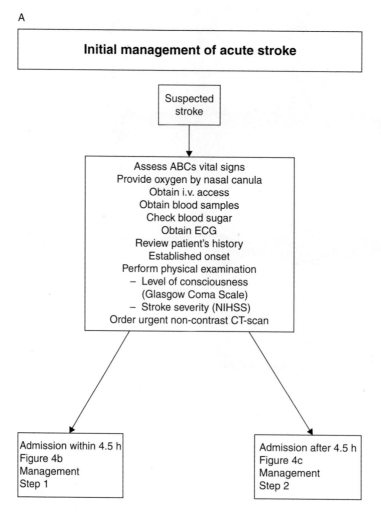

Figure 4(A). Initial management of acute stroke.

either need immediate treatment during the diagnostic procedure itself or after previous magnetic resonance angiography (MRA)/computed tomography angiography (CTA)/ultrasound studies have suggested interventional rather than surgical or conservative therapy planning. MRA and modern ultrasonography have overtaken large domains of conventional angiography and further technical and software development for refined analysis and online investigation will demonstrate preferential use and utility of such techniques in early ischemic stroke monitoring.

However, in patients with hemorrhagic strokes and subarachnoid hemorrhage (SAH) that form 15%–20% of all stroke cases, conventional angiography continues to represent the gold standard for diagnosis, and is increasingly used for

B

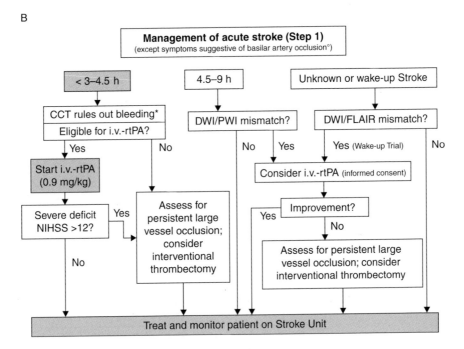

Figure 4(B). Management of acute stroke (Step 1).

Gray = Highlighted, are the only evidence-based treatment options of acute ischemic stroke.
° = Patients with clinical signs of basilar artery occlusion should be treated with i.v. r-tPA as soon as possible, and in individual cases, up to 12 h after onset. In case of subsequent acute worsening, additional intra-arterial thrombolysis/thrombectomy can be considered.
* = Some institutions perform vascular and/or perfusion imaging using CT or MRI in patients presenting within the 3–4.5 h time window (according to national approval), and in selected patients before thrombolysis to identify potential candidates for bridging therapy early on. This approach may lead to a delay of i.v. r-tPA administration; the benefit from thrombolysis, however, has been shown to be greater if started within 90 min after onset. Assessing for large vessel occlusion should be done preferably after the start of thrombolytic therapy.

therapeutic interventions (e.g., coiling of aneurysms) along with neurosurgical approaches.

Cardiovascular investigations on site and in close cooperation within the stroke team taking care of acute stroke patients are important for three major reasons: first, cerebral injury may force cardiac damage, even in patients without pre-existing cardiac disease; second, brain attacks may be cardioembolic in about 20%–30% of the cases; and third, more than half of vascular patients may have coexisting coronary artery disease, and the risk of coronary events with long-term follow-up exceeds the risk of cerebrovascular recurrences. While the last two

C

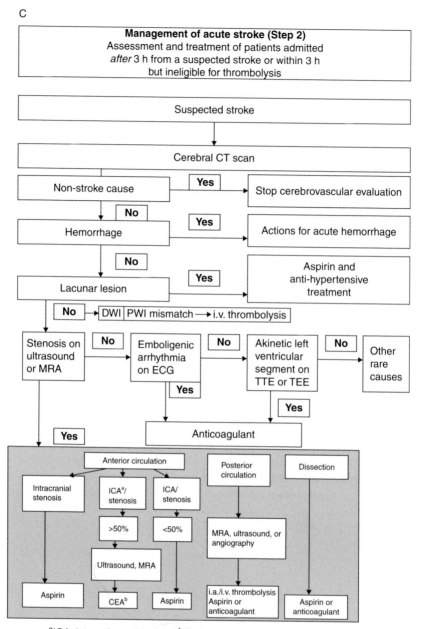

^aICA, internal carotid artery; ^bCEA, carotid endarterectomy

Figure 4(C). Management of acute stroke (Step 2).

reasons are well considered commonly, the first is debated still; knowledge of the pathophysiology of the autonomic system and the increasing number of patients with cerebral death as a possible donor for heart transplantations suggest that the cardiac consequences of cerebral damage is underestimated by far. ECG monitoring has identified numbers of life-threatening ventricular arrhythmias in stroke patients treated on stroke units with continuous ECG monitoring, and consequent treatment has rescued many of them from acute, formerly suspected "stroke death." Acute cerebral injury may cause myocardial damage, which can be documented by two-dimensional echocardiography, serum markers, and myocardial necrosis; the clinical relevance of this is uncertain at present. Possible triggers of ventricular arrhythmia are hypoglycemia, hypoxia, autonomic nervous system imbalance, and Q–T prolongation; some of them can be identified promptly and treated adequately.

Sources of cardioembolic stroke, whether from coexisting cardiovascular or cardiac diseases, need to be diagnosed early and treated immediately to improve late prognosis, because of the coexistence of cerebrovascular and cardiovascular diseases in almost every second patient. A brain attack can be considered a "warning sign" for future coronary events, and therefore, should be of utmost importance in the network of secondary prevention.

A lumbar puncture for CSF analysis is not necessary in the regular patient who presents with cerebrovascular disease; however, it may be indicated if intracranial hemorrhages are suspected (parenchymal and SAHs as well as cerebral venous thrombosis [CVT]), or if forms of isolated angiitis or systemic vasculitis with central nervous system (CNS) involvement are considered. Biomarkers indicating neuronal damage, inflammatory reactions, apoptosis, or poststroke reorganization tissue-associated activities (e.g., superoxide dismutase) increasingly are targets of scientific interest; however, whether taken from the CSF or from the blood, so far they have failed to influence diagnosis (ischemia vs. hemorrhage separation) and therapeutic decisions (staging of acute stroke development within 72 h) directly. Only a small number of laboratory tests (Figure 5) belong to the routine workup of stroke patients; a second group of tests is available to detect rare conditions, such as coagulation abnormalities, antiphospholipid syndromes, vasculitis, and hyperviscosity syndromes in selected patients. A third, very heterogeneous group of laboratory tests still awaits validation for its clinical usefulness, but at present, is considered as experimental.

The history of George Frederick Handel's stroke may guide us on rehabilitation after stroke, reminding us about the enormous capacity of brain plasticity. Once acute stroke treatment and monitoring on the stroke unit is terminated, continuous physical therapy to improve functional reorganization may be necessary, at least in some patients with good prognosis according to very recent but few fMRI and clinical studies, and often for reintegration in family and local social environments. This issue has not been investigated adequately scientifically, despite huge amounts of money spent on rehabilitation compared to acute stroke treatment costs and secondary prevention measures.

Biological System	Test	Compartment	Method	Significance	Current clinical value
Glucose metabolism	Glucose (fasting, tolerance) HbA1c	Blood, urine, plasma	Hexokinase method chromatography	Vascular risk factor, diagnostic	Routine
Lipid metabolism	Cholesterol, triglycerides HDL/LDL-cholesterol	Blood	Enzymatic and precipitation techniques	Vascular risk factor	Routine
	Lp(a)	Blood	ELISA	Vascular risk factor	Routine
Methionine metabolism	Homocyst(e)ine	Blood, urine	HPLC	Diagnostic	Selected conditions
Antithrombotic systems	AT III, protein C, protein S	Plasma	Chromogenic assays, coagulometry	Diagnostic	Selected conditions
Coagulation and fibrinolysis	Prothrombin time, aPTT	Blood	Coagulometry, photometry	Therapy monitoring	Routine
	FM, FpA, TAT, F1+2 D-dimer, B-β-peptide	Plasma	ELISA	Pathogenic	Selected conditions
Systemic host defense	ESR, WBC, CRP	Blood serum	Westergren, impedance counter method, nephelometry	Investigation of acute phase reaction	Routine
	IL-6, IL-1β, TNF-ὰ sICAM-1, sELAM-1, sL-selectin	Serum Plasma	Nephelometry, ELISA ELISA	Endothelial activation	Selected conditions
Viscosity of blood	Hematocrit, fibrinogen	Blood	Microhematocrit technique, coagulometry	Risk factor, pathophysiological	Routine
	Whole blood, plasma viscosity, cell aggregability	Plasma	Filtration technique, shear-viscosimeter, aggregometer		Experimental
HPA system	Cortisol, ACTH	Plasma	RIA	Pathophysiological Prognostic	Experimental
Immune system	ANA, anti-dsDNA Sm-Ag, Scl-70, ANCA	Serum	Immunofluorescence, RIA	Diagnosis of vasculitis (e.g., SLE)	Selected conditions
	Lupus anticoagulant/ anticardiolipin Abs	Plasma	Coagulometry ELISA	Pathogenetic	Selected conditions
Brain tissue integrity	NSE, S-100 protein	Serum, CSF	RIA	Prognostic	Selected conditions

Figure 5.   Synopsis of biological and immunological tests on cerebrovascular diseases.

Convalescence at the hot baths of Aachen brought George Frederick Handel a considerable improvement.

After a week he could drag himself along, after a second week he could move his arm and with enormous "will power" and confidence, he tore himself out of the paralysis of death, for life to be much more fervent than before with every unutterable happiness, as only the recovered know. As "Hallelujah" boomed out for the first time, there was a great cheer…and this was raised again with the last "Amen,"…the jubilation had scarcely filled the room with applause, he simply slipped away, not to thank the people who wanted to thank him, but rather the grace that had endowed this work.

Section 1

Common cases of stroke

Case 1

Woman with aphasia and right-sided numbness

Kristina Szabo

Clinical history

A 70-year-old woman was brought to the emergency room by an ambulance after she developed difficulty communicating, and numbness and weakness of her right arm. Her symptoms fluctuated in severity during a period of more than four hours. Her medical history included hypertension that was not always well controlled and non-insulin-dependent diabetes mellitus.

Examination

Neurological examination upon arrival showed aphasia with impaired naming and reduced verbal fluency, right homonymous hemianopia, and moderate sensorimotor hemiparesis.

Neurological scores: NIHSS 6, mRS 4.

Special studies

Owing to the time from onset that had been witnessed by the patient's daughter, the decision was made to perform acute stroke MRI. MRI showed an acute ischemic lesion in the left posterior cerebral artery (PCA) territory involving the hippocampus with a few additional small scattered lesions in the occipital lobe (Figure 1.1). On MRA, the proximal portion of the left PCA was occluded and correspondingly hypoperfusion was detected in nearly the complete territory supplied by this artery. In a similar approach to stroke in the middle cerebral artery (MCA) territory, this woman was treated with intravenous thrombolysis (IVT) in an extended time window based on the diffusion/perfusion mismatch concept. The door-to-needle time was five hours.

More Case Studies in Stroke, eds. Michael G. Hennerici, Rolf Kern, Louis R. Caplan, and Kristina Szabo. Published by Cambridge University Press. © Cambridge University Press 2014.

Follow-up

Her neurological deficit improved significantly within two hours after therapy and at discharge the homonymous hemianopia had resolved completely (NIHSS 1). Follow-up imaging showed only minimal growth of lesion size on DWI with partial recanalization of the P1 and P2 segments of the left PCA. Extensive examination did not identify a source of embolism. The fluctuating course and her risk factors made it likely that she had had a pre-existing stenosis of the PCA that became occluded.

Imaging findings

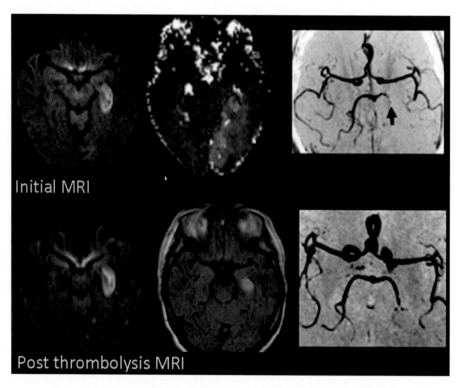

Figure 1.1. MRI before (upper row) and after (bottom row) i.v. thrombolysis: initial MRI shows the ischemic lesion on DWI involving the hippocampus, hypoperfusion on PWI in the left PCA territory and proximal occlusion of the left PCA on MRA. Follow-up MRI lesion on DWI and T2 FLAIR MRI is only slightly larger, while partial vessel recanalization is documented on MRA.

Diagnosis

MRI-guided IVT in PCA territory brain ischemia.

General remarks

Although posterior circulation territory lesions account for about 15%–20% of all ischemic strokes, patients with infarcts in this territory were underrepresented or even excluded from participation in the large clinical trials investigating acute therapy with thrombolysis. The same holds true for clinical trials examining MRI-guided thrombolysis in the posterior circulation based on the PWI/DWI mismatch concept. A higher onset to treatment time in some studies may reflect the unawareness of typical symptoms of posterior circulation territory lesions in the population. The discrepancy between NIHSS and modified Rankin Scale (mRS) scores is attributable to the known inability of the NIHSS to quantify the specific symptoms of posterior circulation territory lesions adequately, and in turn, physicians might hesitate to pursue thrombolysis. In terms of potential benefits and risks of thrombolysis, however, these studies have shown no difference between posterior and anterior circulation territory lesions.

Special remarks

This case supports the approach to treat patients with PCA stroke with thrombolysis based on the PWI/DWI mismatch concept, as one would in the anterior circulation. Studies have shown that mismatch MRI identifies very comparable constellations as in MCA stroke. Therapy enhances the chance of a favorable clinical outcome in these patients. It is worthwhile to note that this case occurred before the ECASS-III trial results led to the extension of the three-hour time window to 4.5 hours. Today, faced with a similar patient and given the remaining time of 30 minutes (presentation was at four hours), we might as well have performed "ultrafast" CT-based thrombolysis.

SUGGESTED READING

Breuer L, Huttner HB, Jentsch K, et al. Intravenous thrombolysis in posterior cerebral artery infarctions. *Cerebrovasc Dis* 2011; **31**: 448–54.

Förster A, Gass A, Kern R, et al. MR imaging-guided intravenous thrombolysis in posterior cerebral artery stroke. *Am J Neuroradiol* 2011; **32**: 419–21.

Pagola J, Ribo M, Alvarez-Sabin J, et al. Thrombolysis in anterior versus posterior circulation strokes: timing of recanalization, ischemic tolerance, and other differences. *J Neuroimaging* 2011; **21**(2): 108–12.

Sato S, Toyoda K, Uehara T, et al. Baseline NIH Stroke Scale score predicting outcome in anterior and posterior circulation strokes. *Neurology* 2008; **70**: 2371–7.

Searls DE, Pazdera L, Korbel E, Vysata O, Caplan LR. Symptoms and signs of posterior circulation ischemia in the New England Medical Center posterior circulation registry. *Arch Neurol* 2012; **69**(3): 346–51.

Dysarthria and hemiparesis

Martin Griebe

Clinical history

A 64-year-old man presented with the acute onset of a speech disturbance, facial palsy, and moderate weakness of the left arm and leg 75 minutes after symptom onset. Except for a history of heavy smoking (45 pack–years), no vascular risk factors were present. ECG and laboratory tests were normal.

Examination

This alert patient had a moderately severe pure motor hemiparesis on the left with facial palsy and moderate dysarthria, constituting a typical lacunar syndrome.

Neurological scores: NIHSS 6, Barthel 40, GCS 15.

Special studies

MRI was performed as the primary stroke imaging. On DWI, a faintly hyper-intense subcortical, paraventricular acute ischemic lesion was detectable that corresponded well with the clinical syndrome (Figure 2.1A). T2-weighted fluid-attenuated inversion recovery (FLAIR) did not show the acute infarct at this stage, but did demonstrate mild to moderate chronic white matter lesions (Figure 2.1B). The intracranial vessels had normal signal on MRA.

Based on these findings, acute systemic thrombolytic therapy was performed 130 minutes after symptom onset. The patient recovered completely within the first day on the stroke unit (NIHSS 0, Barthel 100, GCS 15). No further risk factors or competing etiologies were identified (testing included a three-day Holter-ECG, extra- and transcranial duplex sonography, and transthoracic echocardiography [TTE]). According to the phenotypic classification (ASCOD score: A0 S1 C0 O9 D0), small-vessel stroke was assumed to be the most likely etiology.

More Case Studies in Stroke, eds. Michael G. Hennerici, Rolf Kern, Louis R. Caplan, and Kristina Szabo. Published by Cambridge University Press. © Cambridge University Press 2014.

Ten hours after thrombolytic therapy on follow-up MRI, the acute ischemic lesion had a markedly reduced volume compared to the initial MRI (0.3 ml versus 1.5 ml) being, for the most part, reversible (Figure 2.1C and 2.1D; FLAIR image was blurred due to motion artifacts).

Imaging findings

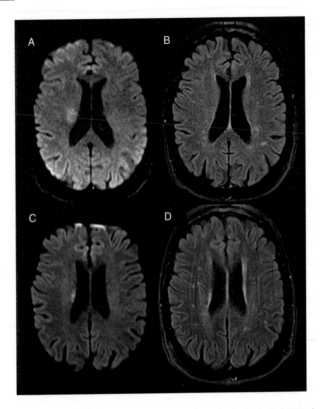

Figure 2.1. MRI before (A, B) and after (C, D) i.v. thrombolysis. Initial MRI shows the faintly hyperintense ischemic lesion on DWI adjacent to the right lateral ventricle but without a T2 correlate. After thrombolysis with clinical recovery, the final lesion size on DWI and T2-weighted FLAIR is considerably smaller.

Diagnosis

Lacunar stroke syndrome with lacunar ischemic lesion, showing marked lesion regression and extensive clinical improvement after thrombolysis.

General remarks

Lacunar stroke represents approximately 25% of all ischemic strokes and has been defined traditionally–on the basis of early neuropathological findings of chronic lacunar lesions–as an acute ischemic stroke caused by occlusion of a single penetrating artery leading to typically located infarcts. Even though it is considered commonly to be a less severe subtype, 30% of patients remain affected by physical disability. Five classical lacunar stroke syndromes have been defined: pure motor stroke, pure sensory stroke, dysarthria/clumsy hand syndrome, ataxic hemiparesis, and sensorimotor stroke. These can be reliably identified based on a thorough clinical examination. Many but by no means all acute lacunar strokes present with one of these five main clinical lacunar stroke syndromes. As many as 20% of patients with a lacunar stroke syndrome are found eventually to be caused by non-lacunar lesions, such as stenosis in the parent arteries that give rise to the penetrating arteries that supply the area of infarction.

Because many lacunar stroke deficits clear rapidly, it is uncertain whether regression was related to the thrombolysis. No trial has investigated the effectiveness, or lack thereof, of i.v. r-tPA in these patients. In the National Institute of Neurological Disorders and Stroke (NINDS) trial, which has been cited often as supporting the effectiveness of r-tPA in all stroke subgroups, there was no important difference in outcome in the groups with varying etiologies, but the quick entry and absence of vascular and cardiac imaging made the clinical diagnosis of stroke etiology and mechanism tentative at best. A committee that reviewed the NINDS results reported that the stroke subtype findings were not valid. A recent abstract indicated that lacunar stroke patients did equally well with or without i.v. thrombolysis. It must be pointed out that because the region of infarction in lacunar strokes is small, there is little if any risk of brain hemorrhage in the area of infarction after r-tPA treatment. For this reason, until more data is available, some neurologists choose to administer i.v. r-tPA in these patients.

Special remarks

A reversal of a stroke lesion in DWI–which is commonly supposed to be the correlate of irreversibly damaged tissue–has been reported repeatedly, yet mostly on the basis of case-reports. The only two systematic studies report divergent prognostic conclusions: the first stating a lesion reversal as a predictor of excellent recovery; in the second, it was not associated with a functional improvement and predicted new (small) embolic lesions.

SUGGESTED READING

Albach FN, Brunecker P, Usnich T, et al. Complete early reversal of diffusion-weighted imaging hyperintensities after ischemic stroke is mainly limited to small embolic lesions. *Stroke* 2013; **44**: 1043–8.

Bamford J, Sandercock P, Jones L, Warlow C. The natural history of lacunar infarction: the Oxfordshire community stroke project. *Stroke* 1987; **18**: 545–51.

Griebe M, Fischer E, Kablau M, et al. Thrombolysis in patients with lacunar stroke is safe: an observational study. *J Neurol* 2014; **261**(2): 405–11.

Ingall TJ, O'Fallon WM, Asplund K, et al. Findings from the reanalysis of the NINDS tissue plasminogen activator for acute ischemic stroke treatment trial. *Stroke* 2004; **35**: 2418–24.

Labeyrie MA, Turc G, Hess A, et al. Diffusion lesion reversal after thrombolysis: an MR correlate of early neurological improvement. *Stroke* 2012; **43**: 2986–91.

Lahoti S, Gokhale S, Caplan LR, et al. Thrombolysis in ischemic stroke with no arterial occlusion: a Multicenter Multinational Retrospective Study. *Neurology* 2013; S52.003.

Norrving B. Long-term prognosis after lacunar infarction. *Lancet Neurol* 2003; **2**: 238–45.

Yamada R, Yoneda Y, Kageyama Y, Ichikawa K. Reversal of large ischemic injury on hyper-acute diffusion MRI. *Case Rep Neurol* 2012; **4**: 177–80.

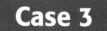

Case 3

From vertigo to coma

Angelika Alonso

Clinical history

A 77-year-old woman presented with vertigo, blurred vision, and hemisensory loss that had started 8.5 hours before admission. She reported blood pressure levels above 200 mmHg over the last 24 hours, and the initially suspected diagnosis was a hypertensive crisis. Lowering of blood pressure in the emergency room, however, did not lead to symptom amelioration. Within another 2.5 hours her symptoms progressed to a state of coma.

Two weeks before this event, she had discontinued one year of oral anti-coagulation treatment following deep vein thrombosis (DVT) and pulmonary embolism.

Examination

Neurological examination on admission showed mild dysarthria and left hemisensory loss. A few hours later, the patient had severe dysarthria, dysphagia, and progressive loss of consciousness, together with rapidly evolving sensorimotor tetraparesis.

Special studies

As posterior circulation stroke was suspected, MRI was ordered and showed an occlusion of the basilar artery with extensive hyperacute ischemic lesions in the brainstem and cerebellum (Figure 3.1).

After confirmation of the basilar artery occlusion, we immediately started i.v. thrombolysis with recombinant r-tPA at a dosage of 0.9 mg/kg body weight about 11 hours after symptom onset, followed by i.v. administration of the GpIIb/IIIa antagonist tirofiban over 48 hours. Clinically, the patient regained consciousness within six hours after thrombolysis, and the neurological deficit markedly improved over the following days. At discharge, the patient had only slight sensorimotor deficits, mild dysarthria, and a skew deviation.

More Case Studies in Stroke, eds. Michael G. Hennerici, Rolf Kern, Louis R. Caplan, and Kristina Szabo. Published by Cambridge University Press. © Cambridge University Press 2014.

Imaging findings

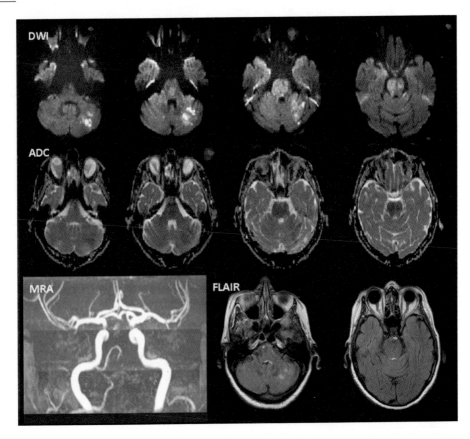

Figure 3.1. DWI shows extensive hyperacute ischemic lesions in the brainstem and cerebellum. Note the marked signal reduction of the pons in the corresponding ADC images and only small regions of cerebellar T2 hyperintensity on FLAIR. On MRA, there is no signal in the basilar artery or the left VA. The right VA appears hypoplastic.

Follow-up

Follow-up MRI on day 1 (Figure 3.2) displayed recanalization of the basilar artery and ischemia in both cerebellar hemispheres. Ischemic lesions in the brainstem were clearly improved on DWI and possibly explain her recovery.

Taking account of her medical history with DVT, we performed TEE to screen for right-to-left shunt. TEE verified a PFO °II, with concomitant atrial septum aneurysm. An intracardiac thrombus could not be detected.

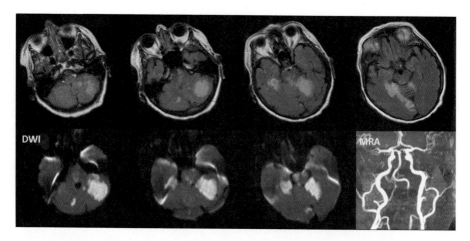

Figure 3.2. Follow-up MRI on day 1 shows recanalization of the basilar artery and the left VA. While cerebellar lesions and a territorial acute ischemic lesion in the right PCA now is strongly DWI- and T2 hyperintense, the brainstem lesions are clearly regressive on DWI.

Neurological scores

At admission:	NIHSS 2, mRS 1, GCS 15.
At start i.v. thrombolysis:	NIHSS 21, mRS 5, GCS 5.
Day 1:	NIHSS 10, mRS 5, GCS 15.
After 1 month:	NIHSS 3, mRS 1, GCS 15.

Diagnosis

Basilar artery occlusion.

General remarks

This patient had an intracranial vertebral artery (VA) occlusion that extended into the basilar artery. Her contralateral VA was hypoplastic. It is not entirely clear if the occlusion was due to embolism from the PFO/atrial septal aneurysm or formed *in situ* within the VA because of hypercoagulability. She had had a DVT and had been on anticoagulants that were stopped before the stroke. The optimal treatment of basilar artery occlusion still is a matter of debate. The primary goal is early recanalization as it is associated with reduced mortality and improved outcome. To date, RCTs comparing primary IVT and IAT are lacking. A recently published prospective, observational registry failed to prove unequivocal superiority of IAT over IVT. At present, the most discussed approach to promote recanalization is a "bridging" concept, combining initial intravenous treatment and subsequent intra-arterial management. However, reliable data on safety and efficacy of combined IVT/IAT are not available yet.

Special remarks

The GpIIb/IIIa antagonist tirofiban has been used widely for the treatment of acute coronary syndrome in combination with heparin and aspirin. The use of tirofiban in the management of acute ischemic stroke within a time window of 3–22 hours after symptom onset has been investigated recently. Treatment with tirofiban was safe and might be favorable in long-term outcome. In basilar artery occlusion, several case series report on combined treatment protocols with tirofiban and IAT. General recommendations for the use of tirofiban cannot be made thus far.

CURRENT REVIEW

Mattle HP, Arnold M, Lindsberg PJ, Schonewille WJ, Schroth G. Basilar artery occlusion. *Lancet Neurol* 2011; **10**(11): 1002–14.

SUGGESTED READING

Schonewille WJ, Wijman CA, Michel P, et al. BASICS study group. Treatment and outcomes of acute basilar artery occlusion in the Basilar Artery International Cooperation Study (BASICS): a prospective registry study. *Lancet Neurol* 2009; **8**(8): 724–30.

Siebler M, Hennerici MG, Schneider D, et al. Safety of tirofiban in acute ischemic stroke: the SaTIS trial. *Stroke* 2011; **42**(9): 2388–92.

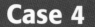

Laughing and crying without apparent reason

Angelika Alonso

Clinical history

A 45-year-old woman of Turkish origin was brought to hospital by her relatives. They reported that they noticed that the patient had a personality change during the past week. She appeared to be either "absent" and showed a limited responsiveness to the surrounding world, or euphoric. Repeatedly, she would start to laugh or cry without any reason. Furthermore, she had urinated on the sofa involuntarily. The symptoms began after a severe family argument, and the relatives suspected a reactive psychological disorder.

Examination

Clinical examination revealed that she was slow to respond to queries or directions and she was disoriented to time, but there were no visual, sensory, motor, or reflex abnormalities.

Neurological scores: NIHSS 1, mRS 2, Barthel 100.

Special studies

DWI identified a large infarction in the left anterior cerebral artery (ACA) territory with inclusion of the superior frontal gyrus and the corpus callosum (Figure 4.1). MRA showed an occlusion of the left ACA. Extracranial Doppler/duplex sonography showed no pathological findings; intracranial sonography confirmed a distal occlusion of the left ACA.

In Holter ECG monitoring, no episodes of atrial fibrillation were recorded, and TEE was normal. Extended screening for laboratory evidence of coagulation disorders revealed high titers of antiphospholipid antibodies, which were confirmed in a second test after six weeks.

More Case Studies in Stroke, eds. Michael G. Hennerici, Rolf Kern, Louis R. Caplan, and Kristina Szabo. Published by Cambridge University Press. © Cambridge University Press 2014.

Imaging findings

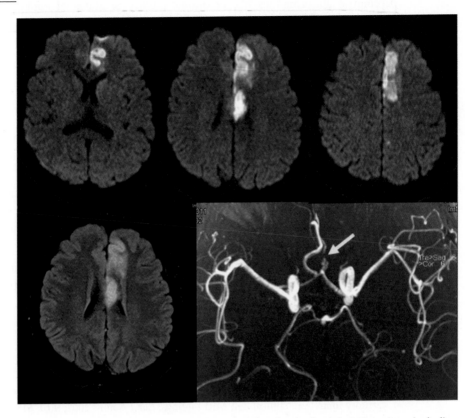

Figure 4.1. DWI and T2 FLAIR images show an extensive infarction in the left ACA territory including the superior frontal gyrus and the corpus callosum. MRA confirms persistent occlusion of the left ACA.

Diagnosis

An acute ACA territory infarct involving the medial frontal lobe in a patient with antiphospholipid antibodies.

General remarks

Behavioral abnormalities are common in ACA territory stroke patients. Mostly following bilateral infarctions of the anterior cingulate gyrus or the head of the caudate nucleus, akinetic mutism with limited responsiveness to stimuli as well as absence of speech and spontaneous movements has been described. In addition, abulia, a state of prolonged but still preserved responsiveness, can occur as a consequence of unilateral lesions of the cingulate gyrus or caudate nucleus.

Lesions involving the medial frontal lobe have been associated with distinct psychiatric abnormalities like emotional lability or states of euphoria.Urinary incontinence is a further typical manifestation of ACA infarction, attributable to affection of the superolateral and medial superior frontal gyrus ("micturition center").

Special remarks

Disinhibition syndromes with euphoric or impulsive behavior result from lesions in the orbitofrontal circuit, involving the orbitofrontal cortex, caudate nucleus, globus pallidus, and thalamus. In addition to focal vascular lesions, traumatic brain injury, frontal lobe tumors, and frontotemporal dementia account for the most common pathoanatomical correlates.

Stroke can be a presenting feature of patients with antiphospholipid antibodies. Brain ischemia is caused by hypercoagulability with arterial and venous occlusions or embolism from associated non-bacterial thrombotic endocarditis. This diagnosis should be considered, especially in young women who have no other stroke risk factors.

CURRENT REVIEW

Kumral E, Bayulkem G, Evyapan D, Yunten N. Spectrum of anterior cerebral artery territory infarction: clinical and MRI findings. *Eur J Neurol* 2002; **9**(6): 615–24.

SUGGESTED READING

Bonelli RM, Cummings JL. Frontal-subcortical circuitry and behavior. *Dialogues Clin Neurosci* 2007; **9**(2): 141–51.

Cervera R, Piette JC, Font J, et al. Antiphospholipid syndrome: clinical and immunologic manifestations and patterns of disease expression in a cohort of 1,000 patients. *Arthritis Rheum* 2002; **46**: 1019–27.

Coull BM, Goodnight SH. Antiphospholipid antibodies, prethrombotic states, and stroke. *Stroke* 1990; **21**: 1370–4.

Levine SR, Kim S, Deegan MI, Welch KMA. Ischemic stroke associated with anticardiolipin antibodies. *Stroke* 1987; **18**: 1101–6.

Roldan JF, Brey RL. Anti-phospholipid antibody syndrome. In Caplan LR (ed.), *Uncommon Causes of Stroke*, 2nd edn. Cambridge: Cambridge University Press, 2008; 263–74.

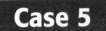

Severe stroke in a 66-year-old man

Angelika Alonso

Clinical history

A 66-year-old-man was found sitting on a park bench with a severe right-sided sensorimotor hemiparesis. Until arrival of the emergency ambulance, his level of consciousness rapidly deteriorated. He was comatose on admission to the hospital. Owing to the lack of brainstem reflexes, he was intubated immediately and mechanically ventilated. His systolic blood pressure at admission was >200 mmHg. Arterial hypertension had been diagnosed years ago; however, he was not taking medication.

Examination

On admission, neurological examination revealed a comatose patient with pre-served spontaneous breathing, no eye opening, and no verbal response. He showed anisocoria with a mydriatic left pupil and preserved pupillary light reflexes. The oculocephalic reflex as well as the corneal reflex was preserved bilaterally. As a response to painful stimuli, he withdrew the left upper limb and flexed the left lower limb while no motor reaction was observed in the right extremities. Monosynaptic reflexes were equal bilaterally, and Babinski's sign was positive on the right side.

Neurological scores: NIHSS 24, mRS 5, GCS 7 deteriorating to 5 rapidly after admission.

Special studies

A cranial CT scan showed an intraparenchymal hemorrhage emerging from the left thalamus with an expansion of approximately 3.5 cm × 3.0 cm × 2.0 cm, corresponding to an estimated volume of about 10 ml according to the formula for

More Case Studies in Stroke, eds. Michael G. Hennerici, Rolf Kern, Louis R. Caplan, and Kristina Szabo. Published by Cambridge University Press. © Cambridge University Press 2014.

ellipsoids (A×B×C/2). The hemorrhage extended into the ventricular system with intraventricular clots in both lateral ventricles and obstruction of the third and fourth ventricle. The subarachnoid space over the brain was considerably narrowed while the lateral ventricles and the temporal horns were widened as a sign of the beginning of an occlusive hydrocephalus (Figure 5.1).

Later management

To prevent the development of severe obstructive hydrocephalus, an external ventricular drain (EVD) was placed in the left lateral ventricle on the day of admission. The patient was transferred to the intensive care unit (ICU), and the mechanical ventilation was continued under anesthesia with midazolam/ sufentanil.

On the following day, the patient had another CT scan that showed a stable intraparenchymal clot volume and slight increase of the perifocal edema. Taking into account the persisting occlusion of the third and fourth ventricle, the patient was treated with intraventricular fibrinolytic therapy and received 1 mg r-tPA every eight hours via the EVD for three days. The follow-up CT scan on day 6 showed complete clearing of blood in the fourth ventricle and a considerably smaller hemorrhage in both lateral ventricles as well as in the third ventricle. The subarachnoid space over the brain and the previously compressed left lateral ventricle were unfolded. The intraparenchymal hemorrhage was unchanged, and the EVD was removed on day 8.

Because of sustained decreased alertness, he could not be extubated, and so the patient was transferred to a rehabilitation center nine days after admission with still-persisting mechanical ventilation. One month after transfer to the rehabili- tation clinic, the patient was weaned from the ventilator successfully. Because of persisting dysphagia, a tracheotomy was performed. He was awake, able to communicate nonverbally, but still in a bedridden state.

Imaging findings

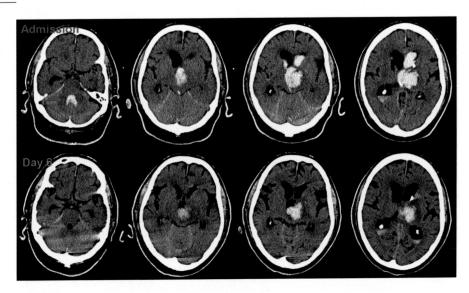

Figure 5.1. Upper row: CT scan on admission, showing an intraparenchymal hemorrhage emerging from the left thalamus with extension into the ventricular system. The fourth ventricle is completely obstructed (arrow), causing the beginning of an occlusive hydrocephalus with widening of the lateral ventricles and their temporal horns. Lower row: follow-up CT scan at day 6. The fourth ventricle is completely cleared from blood (arrow), and the intraventricular hemorrhages in the lateral and third ventricles are smaller. The tip of the external ventricular drain is located in the frontal horn of the left lateral ventricle (*); the widening of the ventricles is clearly improved. The intraparenchymal hemorrhage is stable without any signs of rebleeding.

Diagnosis

Hypertensive hemorrhage starting from the right thalamus, with extension into the ventricular system and obstructive hydrocephalus.

General remarks

The prognosis for patients with large basal ganglionic and thalamic hemorrhages usually is considered to be poor, with a high mortality rate of >40% in the first year and poor functional outcome in the survivors. Main predictors of a negative outcome are large hematoma size, old age, and initially low GCS score. Additionally, an extension of the bleeding into the ventricular system as well as obstructive hydrocephalus further worsens the prognosis. Placement of an EVD has been shown to be effective in reducing elevated intracranial pressure, thus preventing secondary ischemia due to reduced cerebral perfusion pressure. Despite the common use of EVDs in neurointensive care, there is no consensus on the optimal time for treatment. While some authors only require imaging evidence of occlusive hydrocephalus, clinical deterioration is considered to be a precondition for EVD placement by others.

Special remarks

Recently, the effect of intraventricular fibrinolysis on the resolution of intraventricular hemorrhage has been evaluated in several clinical studies. Preliminary results indicate accelerated clot lysis as well as a reduced need for EVD changes or permanent shunting in patients treated with r-tPA via EVD. The ongoing multicenter, double-blind, randomized, placebo-controlled CLEAR III study aims to determine if rapid removal of intraventricular clots with low-dose r-tPA can improve the functional outcome of patients after six months compared to subjects treated only with the best medical care. Many centers already implement intraventricular fibrinolyis off-label, taking account of the CLEAR III inclusion criteria such as a stable intraparenchymal hemorrhage of no more than 30 ml as well as occlusion of the third and/or fourth ventricle.

SUGGESTED READING

Huttner HB, Köhrmann M, Berger C, Georgiadis D, Schwab S. Influence of intraventricular hemorrhage and occlusive hydrocephalus on the long-term outcome of treated patients with basal ganglia hemorrhage: a case-control study. *J Neurosurg* 2006; **105**(3): 412–17.

Huttner HB, Tognoni E, Bardutzky J, et al. Influence of intraventricular fibrinolytic therapy with rt-PA on the long-term outcome of treated patients with spontaneous basal ganglia hemorrhage: a case-control study. *Eur J Neurol* 2008; **15**(4): 342–9.

Liliang PC, Liang CL, Lu CH, et al. Hypertensive caudate hemorrhage prognostic predictor, outcome, and role of external ventricular drainage. *Stroke* 2001; **32**(5): 1195–200.

Webb AJ, Ullman NL, Mann S, et al. Resolution of intraventricular hemorrhage varies by ventricular region and dose of intraventricular thrombolytic: the clot lysis: evaluating accelerated resolution of IVH (CLEAR IVH) Program. *Stroke* 2012; **43**(6): 1666–8.

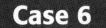

Case 6

Right hemispheric stroke in a young man

Micha Kablau

Clinical history

A 34-year-old right-handed man was hospitalized with right MCA territorial stroke due to dissection of the proximal internal carotid artery (ICA) on the right with complete vessel occlusion and embolic occlusion of an M2 branch of the MCA (Figure 6.1). On follow-up imaging, recanalization of the MCA was shown while the right ICA remained occluded (Figure 6.2).

Clinical course

Despite good neurological improvement within the first two weeks after stroke (NIHSS=2, mRS=3), the patient had persisting affective and cognitive abnormalities. He withdrew from social interactions, and rarely spoke. Not being able to verbalize his feelings, he gave the impression of being depressed. On detailed neuropsychological assessment, he had decreased initiative, motivation, and activity, and reduced ability to persevere with goal-directed activities. While motor and tactile symptoms of neglect improved, reduced visual-constructive abilities persisted. Standardized tests showed executive dysfunctions with reduction of cognitive flexibility and problems in developing and pursuing strategies for problem solution and concept building. The patient was treated with a serotonin-specific reuptake inhibitor (SSRI) and referred to a rehabilitation unit.

More Case Studies in Stroke, eds. Michael G. Hennerici, Rolf Kern, Louis R. Caplan, and Kristina Szabo. Published by Cambridge University Press. © Cambridge University Press 2014.

Imaging findings

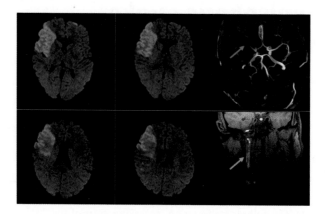

Figure 6.1. DWI (left and middle column) shows a right frontotemporal acute ischemic lesion in the MCA territory. Right top: proximal MCA occlusion (red arrow); right bottom: fat saturated T1-weighted images show hyperintense mural hematoma (orange arrow), indicating ICA dissection.

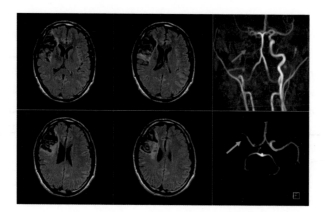

Figure 6.2. Three-month follow-up imaging shows a residual cystic lesion of the infarcted tissue with signs of atrophy in neighboring structures; MRA confirms persisting occlusion of the right ICA (red arrow) and recanalization of the right MCA (orange arrow).

Follow-up

After discharge from rehabilitation two months later, he had improved significantly. Beside slight numbness of the left hand, there were no abnormalities; all neuropsychological test scores had returned to normal.

Diagnosis

Affective disorder after right hemispheric stroke.

General remarks

Up to one third of patients develop depressive symptoms after stroke [1]. The connection of affective disorders and hemispheric neuropsychological defects was first described in the 1970s. Flor-Henry [2] found a lateralized right-hemispheric temporal-limbic dysfunction in patients with affective disorders without any prior indication of an organic cause. The modern concept of poststroke depression does not rely only on the inability of coping with stroke symptoms but implies biological mechanisms such as altered biogenic amine distribution [3] and a lesion location hypothesis especially in the acute phase [4]. Shimoda and Robinson [5] found that during the acute poststroke period, poststroke depression was associated with left anterior lesions. After three to six months, the proximity of the lesion to the frontal pole in both hemispheres rather than the side of the lesion was found to influence the occurrence of poststroke depression.

Patients with frontal lobe and/or caudate nucleus lesions are often abulic. They have decreased initiative and activity but may not feel sad or discouraged or depressed. Abulia is difficult to separate from depression [6].

Special remarks

In our patient, the combination of right hemispheric symptoms and affective disturbances was quite apparent. Although he did not fulfill the criteria for severe depression, this syndrome was diagnosed as a right hemispheric affective disorder. Under antidepressive treatment [7], neuropsychological as well as psychiatric symptoms resolved within two months.

REFERENCES

1. Hackett ML, Yapa C, Parag V, Anderson CS. Frequency of depression after stroke: a systematic review of observational studies. *Stroke* 2005; **36**: 1330–40.
2. Flor-Henry P. Lateralized temporal-limbic dysfunction and psychopathology. *Ann N Y Acad Sci* 1976; **280**: 777–97.
3. Robinson RG, Shoemaker WJ, Schlumpf M, Valk T, Bloom FE. Effect of experimental cerebral infarction in rat brain on catecholamines and behaviour. *Nature* 1975; **22**(255): 332–4.
4. Astrom M, Adolfsson R, Asplund K. Major depression in stroke patients. A three-year longitudinal study. *Stroke* 1993; **24**: 976–82.
5. Shimoda K, Robinson RG. The relationship between poststroke depression and lesion location in long-term follow-up. *Biol Psychiatry* 1999; **45**: 187–92.

6. Ghoshal S, Gokhale S, Rebovich G, Caplan LR. The neurology of decreased activity: abulia. *Rev Neurol Dis* 2011; **8**(3–4): e55–67.

7. Cravello L, Caltagirone C, Spalletta G. The SNRI venlafaxine improves emotional unawareness in patients with post-stroke depression. *Hum Psychopharmacol* 2009; **24**(4): 331–6.

Dysarthria and severe hemiparesis

Valentin Held

Clinical history

A 67-year-old woman presented with an acute onset of dysarthria and severe left-sided hemiparesis. She was admitted to our stroke unit and systemic thrombolysis was administered three hours after onset of symptoms. She recovered promptly with only a slight left-sided facial palsy remaining. Her general history was unrevealing except for arterial hypertension and elevated blood cholesterol.

Examination

Neurological scores

On admission: NIHSS 11, Barthel 20, mRS 5.
After thrombolysis: NIHSS 2, Barthel 100, mRS 1.
On discharge: NIHSS 1, Barthel 100, mRS 1.

Special studies

While a dense-media sign was visible on CT before thrombolysis, extra- and intracranial Doppler and duplex sonography as well as MRA after thrombolysis did not show any relevant stenosis or occlusion. DWI showed acute ischemic stroke affecting the right lenticular nucleus, as well as the head and body of the caudate nucleus (Figure 7.1). ECG monitoring and echocardiography failed to identify a cardiogenic source of embolism.

More Case Studies in Stroke, eds. Michael G. Hennerici, Rolf Kern, Louis R. Caplan, and Kristina Szabo. Published by Cambridge University Press. © Cambridge University Press 2014.

Imaging findings

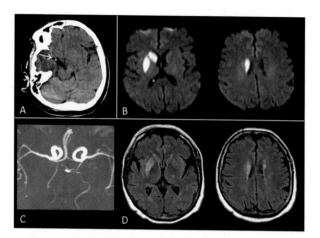

Figure 7.1. (A): CT before thrombolysis suggests a dense media sign on the right (arrow). (B,D): DWI and T2-FLAIR images performed after thrombolysis show an acute ischemic lesion of the right putamen and caudate nucleus, sparing the internal capsule. (C): on MRA, the right MCA seems somewhat more prominent than the left – a possible subtle sign of recanalization.

Diagnosis

Embolic lenticular infarction of unknown etiology–with excellent resolution after thrombolysis.

General remarks

Hemiparesis and dysarthria are the most common symptoms of putaminal infarction. As it is involved in many higher functions via the frontal-subcortical circuits, other symptoms may be prevalent as well. These include symptoms usually linked to cortical ischemia, such as aphasia. Depending on the exact structures involved, movement disorders such as dystonia, hemiparkinsonism, and hemiballism may evolve as well. While the prognosis may be good when only the putamen is involved, an involvement of the internal capsule, as is common, is usually predictive of more persistent motor dysfunction. When the anterior limb of the capsule is infarcted, the weakness may be slight. According to the structures involved, striatocapsular infarction has been suggested as an alternative name, while "giant lacune" puts emphasis on the morphology and also the mechanism when several large lenticulostriate arterial branches are occluded.

The putamen is supplied by the lenticulostriate arteries stemming from the M1 segment of the MCA. Occlusion of the proximal MCA can lead to an ischemic stroke of the entire territory. When there is good collateralization via meningeal arteries, the distal parts of the territory are spared. At times, the perfusion delivered by collateral vessels is inadequate to maintain metabolism and brain tissue within the previous penumbra becomes infarcted.

Special remarks

Recovery from stroke is presumed to be a function of a cerebral network. While study results are contradictory, some have shown that small vessel disease increases the susceptibility to infarct growth, and thus have provided a first mechanism explaining how it may cause poor recovery from stroke. The striato-capsular region is an area of high connectivity, and therefore, seemingly ideal to test the hypothesis that the extent of small vessel disease, via a disturbance of the cerebral network, might affect the course in acute stroke. Recent data found that the severity of small vessel disease was a predictor of poor outcome and recovery in striatocapsular stroke, independent of age or comorbidity. The excellent out-come in this case may be multifactorial: not only was thrombolysis performed early but, in addition, there was only minimal small vessel disease.

SUGGESTED READING

Ay H, Arsava E, Rosand J, et al. Severity of leukoaraiosis and susceptibility to infarct growth in acute stroke. *Stroke* 2008; **39**: 1409–13.

Giroud M, Lemesle M, Madinier G, Billiar T, Dumas R. Unilateral lenticular infarcts: radiological and clinical syndromes, aetiology, and prognosis. *BMJ* 1997; **63**(5): 611.

Held V, Szabo K, Bäzner H, Hennerici MG. Chronic small vessel disease affects clinical outcome in patients with acute striatocapsular stroke. *Cerebrovasc Dis* 2012; **33**(1): 86–91.

Russmann H, Vingerhoets F, Ghika J, Maeder P, Bogousslavsky J. Acute infarction limited to the lenticular nucleus: clinical, etiologic, and topographic features. *Arch Neurol* 2003; **60**(3): 351–5.

van Overbeek EC, Knottnerus ILH, van Oostenbrugge RJ. Disappearing hyperdense middle cerebral artery sign is associated with striatocapsular infarcts on follow-up CT in ischemic stroke patients treated with intravenous thrombolysis. *Cerebrovasc Dis* 2010; **30**(3): 285–9.

Section 2

Uncommon cases of stroke

Case 8

Stroke in a 12-year-old girl

Manuel Bolognese

Clinical history

A 12-year-old girl was carried into the pediatric emergency room by her father. The father reported that she turned cyanotic and collapsed while playing football. The family reported a shivering of both arms and legs.

Examination

On examination, the girl had a severe left hemispheric syndrome with global aphasia, conjugated gaze deviation to the left, severe hemiparesis with Babinski sign, and hemisensory loss on the right side. She was drowsy but arousable, and her vital signs were normal.

Neurological scores: NIHSS 18, mRS 5, Barthel 0, GCS 10.

Special studies

Cerebral MRI showed an acute ischemic stroke (Figure 8.1A, B) involving the insula, the lentiform nucleus, and the head of the caudate nucleus. MRA showed occlusion of the distal M3 branches of the left MCA with irregular contrasting of the left proximal MCA and distal ICA (Figure 8.1D). MRI perfusion imaging revealed an extended perfusion deficit beyond the territory of the diffusion impairment in the cortical areas of the MCA territory (Figure 8.1C). Laboratory studies including an extended coagulation profile, screening for vasculitis, and analysis of CSF yielded normal results. TTE and TEE also showed no abnormalities.

Cervical and transcranial duplex sonography gave indirect signs of a distal stenosis in the carotid siphon with decreased maximum systolic flow velocity in the left ICA and retrograde flow in the left proximal ACA segment, indicating a hemodynamic compensation from the right to the left anterior circulation.

More Case Studies in Stroke, eds. Michael G. Hennerici, Rolf Kern, Louis R. Caplan, and Kristina Szabo. Published by Cambridge University Press. © Cambridge University Press 2014.

Digital subtraction angiography confirmed the distal ICA and proximal MCA stenosis with typical constrictions like "strings of beads," characteristic for fibro-muscular dysplasia (Figure 8.1E).

Follow-up

Around five hours after onset of the symptoms, we treated the child with IVT, based on DWI/PWI mismatch criteria. Follow-up MRI showed a recanalization of the distal MCA branches with no further ischemic transformation of the initially hypoperfused area, while the distal ICA and proximal MCA obstruction persisted. We treated the patient with oral anticoagulation and intensive physical-, ergo-, and speech therapy. The patient was discharged from our hospital to a rehabilitation center after four weeks (NIHSS 8, mRS 4 at discharge). We saw her again in our outpatient department after another three months with a moderate right spastic hemiparesis and mild residual aphasia. She was able to walk without any help (NIHSS 5, mRS 3).

Imaging findings

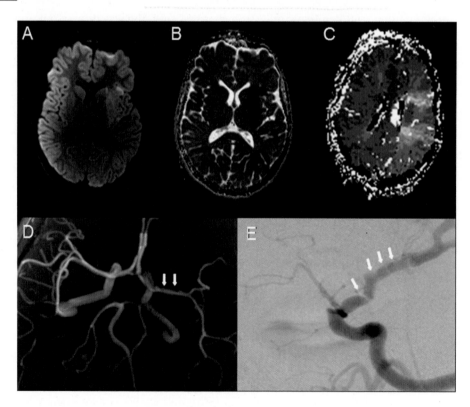

Figure 8.1. (A,B): DWI scan (A) and corresponding ADC-map (B) showing acute ischemic stroke of the left lentiform nucleus, head of the caudate nucleus, and the insular cortex. (C): PWI scan

Diagnosis

Intracranial fibromuscular dysplasia with acute MCA stroke, most likely due to arterioarterial embolization into the distal MCA branches.

General remarks

The incidence of stroke in children is reported to vary from 1.3 to 13.0/100000. There is insufficient data concerning the treatment of acute ischemic stroke in children, both regarding acute reperfusion treatment and the best secondary prevention. Another major problem is the frequent delay in diagnosis of stroke in children, as parents, family members, or doctors rarely assume this diagnosis in pediatric patients as the reason for acute neurological deficits.

Fibromuscular dysplasia is very rare in children, being reported only in a few case studies as a potential cause of ischemic stroke. Most of the time, MRA does not provide sufficient resolution to show the small multi-segmental structural changes of the brain-supplying arteries; thus digital subtraction angiography is needed to confirm the diagnosis. Because fibromuscular dysplasia of the carotid or intracranial arteries often remains asymptomatic, the treatment and prevention concepts are not evidence based, especially not in children. In adults, the abnormal elastic tissue within the fibromuscular dysplastic arteries is associated with hypercontractility and calcium channel blockers, and verapamil, for example, can be therapeutic.

Special remarks

In our patient, we faced the problem of delayed diagnosis of stroke. Because of the collapse and possible convulsions, an epileptic seizure was assumed initially as the most likely diagnosis, and MRI was performed only after some delay. The neurologist was contacted when the state of the young patient did not improve and MRI revealed an acute ischemic stroke.

Caption for Figure 8.1 (*cont.*)
showing delayed contrast bolus arrival in the left MCA territory. D: TOF-angiography with irregular contrasting of the proximal left MCA (arrows). E: Digital subtraction angiography with typical "strings of beads" constrictions of the left distal ICA and left proximal MCA (arrows).

SUGGESTED READING

Amlie-Lefond C, Sébire G, Fullerton HJ. Recent developments in childhood arterial ischemic stroke. *Lancet Neurol* 2008; **7**: 425–35.

Amlie-Lefond C, de Veber G, Chan AK, et al. Use of alteplase in childhood arterial ischaemic stroke: a multicentre, observational, cohort study. *Lancet Neurol* 2009; **8**: 530–6.

Arnold M, Steinlin M, Baumann A, et al. Thrombolysis in childhood stroke: report of 2 cases and review of literature. *Stroke* 2009; **40**: 801–7.

Kirkham F, Sébire G, Steinlin M, Sträter R. Arterial ischaemic stroke in children. Review of the literature and strategies for future stroke studies. *Thromb Haemost* 2004; **92**: 697–706.

Plouin PF, Perdu F, La Batide Alanore A, et al. Fibromuscular dysplasia. *Orphanet J Rare Dis* 2007; **2**: 28.

Rafay MF, Pontigon AM, Chiang J, et al. Delay to diagnosis in acute pediatric arterial ischemic stroke. *Stroke* 2009; **40**: 58–64.

Woman with headache, arthritis, and nausea

Johannes Binder and Kristina Szabo

Clinical history

A 52-year-old woman consulted her family physician due to headaches that were located in the front of the head and affected both sides. In addition, she had felt intermittently nauseated and had vomited several times. She also had noted pain in her jaw when eating. These symptoms had become more frequent and more severe during a period of two weeks. After several episodes of transient shimmering occurred in her right eye she was sent for an MRI of the brain. Additionally, she reported nightly pain in her shoulders and legs, tinnitus, general fatigue, and a weight loss of 8 kg in the previous six months. She had been in three rehabilitation programs due to chronic arthritis. She was referred to our neurology department with multiple acute and subacute ischemic lesions in the posterior inferior cerebellar artery (PICA) territory of the left cerebellum.

Examination

Upon admission she had no neurological deficit. Palpation of the temporal and occipital arteries showed patchy areas of firm vascular walls and absent pulsations. Laboratory tests in the emergency room showed an increase in C-reactive protein (CRP) (15.9 mg/L).

Special studies

Extracranial color-coded ultrasound revealed a high resistance flow profile in both ICAs (L>R; 2 m/s vs. 1.2 m/s). The left VA had a focal stenosis in the V4 segment, while the right VA had concentric, homogeneous, and smooth hypoechogenic mural thickening. The transcranial examination revealed additional stenosis in the left distal MCA (2 m/s). These findings were all confirmed by MRI (Figures 9.1 and 9.2). Blood sedimentation rate was increased to 60 mm in the first hour;

More Case Studies in Stroke, eds. Michael G. Hennerici, Rolf Kern, Louis R. Caplan, and Kristina Szabo. Published by Cambridge University Press. © Cambridge University Press 2014.

other vasculitis parameters were negative. A superficial temporal artery biopsy (Figure 9.3) was performed after the so-called halo sign was found to be present in an ultrasound examination of the temporal artery.

Imaging findings

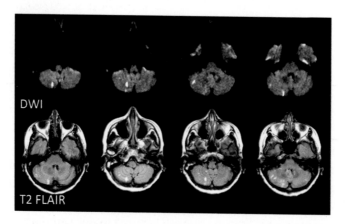

Figure 9.1. DWI and FLAIR images show multiple acute ischemic lesions in the left and one on the border of the right PICA territory. Note that not all T2-hyperintense lesions are strongly visible on DWI, suggesting the presence of additional subacute lesions.

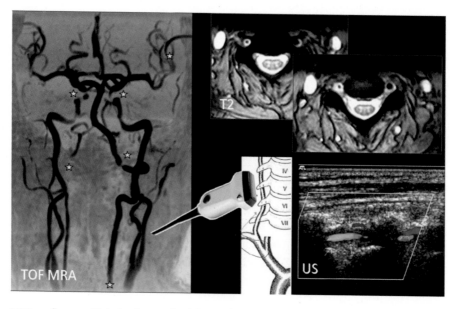

Figure 9.2. MRA confirms multiple focal stenosis of the cerebral arteries (L-MCA, and both distal ICAs, L>R, L-VA) and long-segment narrowing of the right VA. On T2-weighted transverse sections and ultrasound, homogeneous and regular hyperintense/hypoechogenic mural thickening is present.

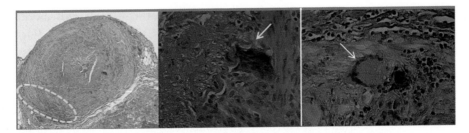

Figure 9.3. Biopsy specimen (H/E stain) of the right temporal artery shows lymphocytic infiltration of the vessel wall (dotted circle), fragmentation of the internal elastic lamina, and large multinucleated cells ("giant cells") (arrows).

Diagnosis

Systemic giant cell arteritis and cerebellar infarction.

Follow-up

The patient received 1000 mg i.v. methylprednisolone for five days, followed by gradual tapering of the dose to 10 mg daily. An evaluation for malignancy was negative. She remained asymptomatic while taking 100 mg aspirin and low-dose corticosteroids even though the vessel findings did not improve during the course of the first 12 months.

General remarks

Giant cell arteritis, also termed temporal or cranial arteritis or Horton disease is a systemic, inflammatory disease affecting branches of the external carotid artery especially, and predominantly the temporal arteries. It is more common in women and occurs after the age of 55 years. Giant cell arteritis commonly is associated with polymyalgia rheumatica. The American College of Rheumatology defined the following criteria for the diagnosis of giant cell arteritis: (1) age 50 years and older, (2) recent onset of localized headache, (3) temporal artery tenderness or decreased temporal artery pulse, (4) ESR of at least 50 mm/h, and (5) abnormal artery biopsy specimen characterized by mononuclear infiltration or granulomatous inflammation. Heterogeneous symptoms resulting from systemic inflammatory disorder include fatigue, fever, weight loss, proximal muscle pain and stiffness, and joint symptoms, especially tenderness of the hip and shoulder. Additional symptoms of involvement of arteries of the head are jaw and tongue claudication, tongue necrosis, tinnitus, diplopia, and reduced visual acuity. If the ophthalmic artery is affected, loss of vision may develop abruptly and needs immediate therapy to prevent irreversible blindness. High-dose corticosteroids must be started if this diagnosis is suspected–in severe cases, even before the biopsy.

Special remarks

An early pathological study examining the pattern of arterial involvement in giant cell arteritis found a very high incidence of severe involvement of the superficial temporal, vertebral, ophthalmic, and posterior ciliary arteries, while the internal carotid, external carotid, and central retinal arteries were severely involved less commonly. Several studies have estimated the incidence of ischemic stroke due to the disease to be around 3%–4%, while in a few cases (about 0.15% in one series)– as in ours–posterior circulation stroke may be the presenting symptom and lead to the diagnosis of giant cell arteritis. It should be kept in mind if concentric, long-segment, increased thickening of the vessel wall of cerebral arteries is detected (homogeneous and regular hyperintense/hypoechogenic mural thickening in MRI [T2-weighted transverse sections] and ultrasound [color-coded duplex ultra-sound]). Depending on the severity of vessel obstruction and individual risk assessment, therapy with aspirin or oral anticoagulation, in addition to cortico-steroids, needs to be considered.

SUGGESTED READING

Gonzalez-Gay MA, Blanco R, Rodriguez-Valverde V, et al. Permanent visual loss and cerebrovascular accidents in giant cell arteritis: predictors and response to treatment. *Arthritis Rheum* 1998; **41**: 1497–504.

Hunder GG, Bloch DA, Michel BA, et al. The American College of Rheumatology 1990 criteria for the classification of giant cell arteritis. *Arthritis Rheum* 1990; **33**(8): 1122–8.

Rüegg S, Engelter S, Jeanneret C, et al. Bilateral vertebral artery occlusion resulting from giant cell arteritis: report of 3 cases and review of the literature. *Medicine* 2003; **82**(1): 1–12.

Wilkinson IM, Russell RW. Arteries of the head and neck in giant cell arteritis. A pathological study to show the pattern of arterial involvement. *Arch Neurol* 1972; **27**(5): 378–91.

Wiszniewska M, Devuyst G, Bogousslavsky J. Giant cell arteritis as a cause of first-ever stroke. *Cerebrovasc Dis* 2007; **24**(2–3): 226–30.

Case 10

Woman with transient sensory disturbance

Kristina Szabo

Clinical history

A 71-year-old woman was admitted to the emergency room because of transient sensory symptoms of the left leg the day before.

Examination

Neurological examination was normal. It was noted that there was no obvious disturbance of memory.

Special studies/imaging findings

Stroke MRI revealed vessel pathology of the P2-segment of the right PCA, with two corresponding acute ischemic lesions found on DWI, namely in the right hippocampus and a small lesion in the splenium of the corpus callosum (Figures 10.1 and 10.2). All investigations for potential sources of embolism were negative. She was treated with aspirin for secondary prophylaxis.

Additional neuropsychological testing revealed impaired nonverbal long-term memory as measured by the Rey–Osterrieth complex figure test. This test analyzes visuographic memory; patients are asked to copy a complex figure accurately and to reproduce it after a delay of three minutes. All other neuropsychological test findings were within the normal range.

More Case Studies in Stroke, eds. Michael G. Hennerici, Rolf Kern, Louis R. Caplan, and Kristina Szabo. Published by Cambridge University Press. © Cambridge University Press 2014.

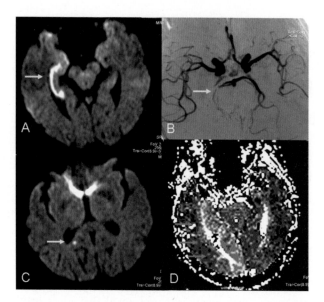

Figure 10.1. DWI shows a hyperintense ischemic lesion in the lateral part of the right hippocampus (A). An additional dot-like lesion is found near the right lateral aspect of the splenium of the corpus callosum (C). On MRA, the stenosis of the P2 segment of the right PCA is visible (B, yellow arrow) corresponding to hypoperfusion with delayed contrast agent arrival on the time-to-peak map (D, red arrows) of the perfusion image.

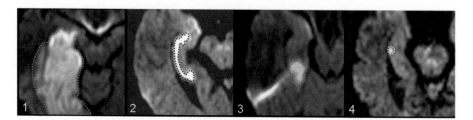

Figure 10.2. Patterns of acute ischemic lesions of the hippocampus on DWI affecting the complete hippocampus (1) and the lateral (2) or dorsal (3) parts of the hippocampal body and tail, and small circumscribed lesions in the lateral hippocampus (4).

Diagnosis

Right hippocampal infarction.

General remarks

Descriptions of acute ischemic stroke lesions affecting the hippocampus and its symptomatology are rare–being mainly descriptions of bilateral ischemic lesions of the hippocampus and accompanying neuropsychological symptoms. In 1900, the Russian neurologist Bechterew described a patient who experienced amnesia related to stroke, while the postmortem study revealed bilateral softening involving the uncus and the Ammon's horn. In 1961, a similar postmortem study of a patient with bilateral infarctions in the PCA territories established stroke as an etiology of acute and, in particular, persistent amnesia. The common feature in all unilateral cases of amnesia related to hippocampal stroke reported after these early studies and based on CT-imaging alone was the involvement of the left hippocampus. In a recent study using DWI for exact lesion description, we found four main patterns of hippocampal lesions in acute stroke, corresponding well to the vascular anatomy of the PCA and its hippocampal branches. Another finding was that we did not see patients with isolated stroke of the hippocampus. This contrasts with other diseases like herpes simplex encephalitis, paraneoplastic limbic encephalitis, or transient global amnesia, which may involve one or both hippocampi predominately or exclusively.

Special remarks

The striking feature of this case is the affection of the hippocampus as a manifestation of acute ischemic stroke in the PCA territory. Neuropsychological examination revealed moderately impaired nonverbal long-term memory. It is important to keep in mind that detailed neuropsychological examination in hippocampal stroke patients might reveal mildly or moderately impaired verbal long-term memory in left hippocampal ischemic lesions and nonverbal long-term memory deficits in right hippocampal ischemic lesions. Both are cognitive areas that may well escape a standard neurological examination in acute stroke patients. This underlines the necessity of a detailed neuropsychological assessment. Although overt cognitive deficits in hippocampal stroke are rare, a study suggests that stroke lesions in the hippocampus may become relevant in the presence of a second pathology like Alzheimer's dementia. The combination of the two pathologies may lead to the unmasking and decompensation of a fragile, compensated functional state and thereby may be important in the physiopathology of mixed vascular dementia and Alzheimer's disease.

SUGGESTED READING

Bechterew W. Demonstration eines Gehirns mit Zerstörung der vorderen und inneren Teile der Hirnrinde beider Schläfenlappen. *Neurologisches Zentralblatt* 1900; **19**: 990–1.

Del Ser T, Hachinski V, Merskey H, Munoz DG. Alzheimer's disease with and without cerebral infarcts. *J Neurol Sci* 2005; **231**(1–2): 3–11.

Förster A, Griebe M, Gass A, et al. Value of diffusion-weighted imaging in differential diagnosis of hippocampal pathologies. *Cerebrovasc Dis* 2012; **33**(2): 104–15.

Szabo K, Förster A, Jäger T, et al. Hippocampal lesion patterns in acute posterior cerebral artery stroke: clinical and MRI findings. *Stroke* 2009; **40**: 2042–5.

Victor M, Angevine JB, Mancall EL, Fisher CM. Memory loss with lesions of hippocampal formation. Report of a case with some remarks on the anatomical basis of memory. *Arch Neurol* 1961; **5**: 244–63.

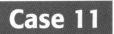

A severe attack of migraine

Marc Wolf

Clinical history

A 43-year-old woman complained about severe right-sided headache and loss of vision to her left. She had a history of migraine with visual aura for over 10 years and was on a prophylactic medication with metoprolole. She reported that she had felt her typical visual disturbances in the left visual field two days ago with severe right-sided hemicrania; however, despite taking nonsteroidal anti-inflammatory drugs (NSAIDs), the visual loss persisted.

Examination

Neurological examination revealed a left homonymous hemianopia. The patient complained about severe right-sided hemicrania (5/10 on the visual analog scale).
Neurological scores: NIHSS 2, Barthel 100, mRS 2.

Special studies

MRI studies showed an acute territorial infarction in the territory of the right PCA on DWI with matching hypoperfusion in dynamic susceptibility contrast perfusion imaging (Figure 11.1). Doppler/duplex sonography of the extra-/intracranial vessels showed slightly elevated flow velocities in the right P2 segment of the PCA. TEE showed no abnormalities, especially no PFO. Perimetric studies of the visual field confirmed homonymous hemianopia in the left visual field.

More Case Studies in Stroke, eds. Michael G. Hennerici, Rolf Kern, Louis R. Caplan, and Kristina Szabo. Published by Cambridge University Press. © Cambridge University Press 2014.

Imaging findings

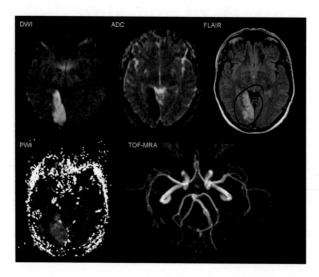

Figure 11.1. DWI (left upper row) shows a territorial PCA infarction with a corresponding hypointense ADC lesion (middle upper row). The infarction is already demarcated on FLAIR imaging (right upper row). PWI shows a hypoperfusion in the ischemic area (left bottom row), TOF-MRA shows a slight rarefication of the distal PCA branches.

Diagnosis

Migrainous infarction in the right PCA territory.

General remarks

Migrainous infarction is a well-defined stroke subtype affecting patients with a known history of migraine. The typical case is characterized by typical visual aura symptoms as known from previous migraine attacks, but persisting over 60 minutes and showing an acute ischemic stroke on neuroimaging. Brainstem and cerebellar infarction can also occur. Other etiologies must be excluded. Migrainous infarction is rare with a prevalence of 0.5%–1.5% of all ischemic strokes; it affects mainly young women with additional cardiovascular risk factors (e.g., oral contraception and smoking) and predominantly occurs in the posterior circulation territory.

Special remarks

Because the occurrence of aura symptoms is quite common in migraineurs, they often seek medical help with some delay if symptoms persist and options for a systemic thrombolytic treatment are missed. Therefore, patients with migraine with aura and additional cardiovascular risk factors should be aware of the potential risk of this rare complication.

SUGGESTED READING

Caplan LR. Migraine and vertebrobasilar ischemia. *Neurology* 1991; **41**: 55–61.

Kurth T, Chabriat H, Bousser MG. Migraine and stroke: a complex association with clinical implications. *Lancet Neurol* 2012; **11**: 92–100.

Laurell K, Artto V, Bendtsen L, et al. Migrainous infarction: a Nordic multicenter study. *Eur J Neurol* 2011; **18**: 1220–6.

Wolf ME, Szabo K, Griebe M, et al. Clinical and MRI characteristics of acute migrainous infarction. *Neurology* 2011; **76**: 1911–17.

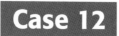

An acute loss of vision

Tilman Menzel

Clinical history and examination

A 71-year-old woman was admitted to the emergency room 3.5 hours after onset of a left homonymous hemianopia. Apart from a slight right frontal hemicrania, clinical neurological and neuro-ophthalmological examination were normal. Cranial CT showed only chronic infarctions in the right frontal MCA- and left PCA-territories, and hence the patient was treated with r-tPA intravenously according to the results of the European Cooperative Acute Stroke Study ECASS-III, unfortunately without improvement of the visual field defects.

The following day, the patient reported acute total loss of vision of her right eye; the left eye still had a hemianopia for the left visual field (Figure 12.1). Although 1.5-Tesla-MRI of the brain did not show any acute lesion in DWI or T2* images, the patient was treated with r-tPA i.v. again, this time with half dosage, but again without any effect on the visual loss.

Neurological scores: NIHSS 2, mRS 2.

Special studies

Because standard MRI of the brain had failed to show any lesion corresponding to the deficit of the visual field suggesting sequential involvement of the right optic tract and optic nerve including the chiasm, a high-resolution 3-Tesla-MRI was performed, which showed an acute DWI- and apparent diffusion coefficient (ADC) lesion in the right optic nerve and chiasm. The neural tissue was hyperintense in T2-weighted imaging and showed an enhancement after contast-agent administration (Figure 12.2).

Ultrasound and a biopsy of the right temporal artery demonstrated unspecific thickening of its intimal layer, but no signs for giant cell arteritis. Doppler- and

More Case Studies in Stroke, eds. Michael G. Hennerici, Rolf Kern, Louis R. Caplan, and Kristina Szabo. Published by Cambridge University Press. © Cambridge University Press 2014.

duplex-sonography as well as MRA showed only mild plaques of the large cerebral arteries.

Laboratory studies were inconclusive: systemic vasculitis or neuritis seemed unlikely (ESR 17 mm/h, CRP normal, ANA 1:320 [N: 0–1:80], ENA [especially DS-DNS and SSA/SSB] and ANCA normal, CSF-ACE normal, syphilis titers negative). However, local atopic inflammation could not be excluded–the screening for anti-cardiolipin and anti-B2-glycoprotein antibodies showed mildly increased titers, while phosphatidylserine antibodies were normal. Rheumatoid factor IgG and IgM were positive.

Total IgE levels were very high with up to 1895 kU/L in the serum (N: 0–120), while total IgG and IgM levels were mildly increased. Mite-specific IgE levels were very high, especially for *Dermatophagoides spp.* In contrast, there was no blood eosinophilia in repeat testing and no clinical or radiological signs indicated pulmonary pathology. The patient's history had no previous asthmatic or other atopic diseases. Lumbar puncture showed no signs of inflammation and was otherwise normal (cell count 1/μl, protein 706 mg/L).

Imaging findings

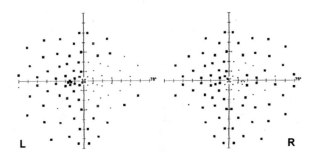

Figure 12.1. Computer-aided perimetry of the patient's visual fields demonstrating the combined homonymous hemianopia to the left of both eyes and amaurosis of the right eye.

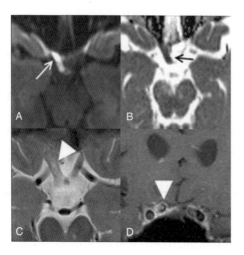

Figure 12.2. (A, B): transverse plane, showing a notable diffusion restriction with a corresponding ADC lesion of the posterior right optic nerve and the right optic chiasm (arrows); (C, D): transverse and coronal planes, respectively, showing a T2-weighted hyperintensity and enhancement of contrast agent in T1-weighted imaging of the posterior right optic nerve and the right optic chiasm (arrowheads).

Diagnosis

Optic nerve ischemia.

General remarks

This case report illustrates important difficulties in patients suspected to have acute cerebral ischemia of the posterior cerebral circulation, who–different from patients with sensorimotor or speech disturbances due to acute stroke or TIAs in the anterior cerebral circulation–are selected for early thrombolysis in emergency units less frequently.

Acute posterior ischemic optic neuropathy (PION) is a rare cause of visual field defects and might have been overlooked more often than reported, in particular if careful and selective MR-based neuroimaging of the optic nerve, chiasm, and tract are not performed. In the acute phase only a few hours after onset, the diagnosis is even more difficult. This is probably why such a subtle lesion, mimicking acute stroke in the territory of the PCA, has not been reported to date. Failure of collateral blood supply within the extensive arterial network from the carotid artery is similarly rare; thus only blockage of small penetrating arteries branching off the intracranial siphon of the carotid artery could account for this highly specific ischemic pattern.

This case strengthens the importance of repeat MRI in patients with persistent visual field defects despite normal acute MRI. Furthermore, high resolution imaging of the visual system should be performed in all cases of ophthalmologically undetermined visual field defects.

Special remarks

Owing to the aforementioned clinical features, MRI, and laboratory results, PION was the most likely diagnosis. Exact epidemiological data being sparse, PIONs are rare diseases with much lower incidences than anterior ischemic optic neuropathies. Like these, PIONs are divided into arteriitic and non-arteriitic types.

A possible differential diagnosis was arteritis limited to intracranial vessels, such as an intracranial granulomatous arteritis or a primary angiitis of the CNS. The good clinical condition and follow-up of our patient, the normal CRP, the near-normal ESR, and the unspecific results of the biopsy of the temporal artery excluded this diagnosis. However, the very high total and mite-specific IgE-titers might suggest a vascular involvement in an atopic inflammation of central nervous tissue, which has come to attention only in recent years but is not well defined as a clinical entity to date.

CURRENT REVIEW

Hayreh SS. Ischemic optic neuropathy. *Prog Retin Eye Res* 2009; **28**(1): 34–62.

SUGGESTED READING

Birnbaum J, Hellmann DB. Primary angiitis of the central nervous system. *Arch Neurol* 2009; **66**(6): 704–9.

Hajj-Ali RA, Calabrese LH. Central nervous system vasculitis. *Curr Opin Rheumatol* 2009; **21**(1): 10–18.

Isobe N, Kira J, Kawamura N, et al. Neural damage associated with atopic diathesis: a nationwide survey in Japan. *Neurology* 2009; **73**(10): 790–7.

vanOverbeeke J, Sekhar L. Microanatomy of the blood supply to the optic nerve. *Orbit* 2003; **22**(2): 81–8.

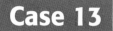

Case 13

Angiography with complications

Alex Förster and Kristina Szabo

Clinical history

A 73-year-old man with suspected coronary artery disease underwent coronary angiography. Toward the end of the angiography he noted double vision and became progressively drowsy. The procedure was stopped and the acute stroke team was informed.

Examination

Upon arrival of the stroke neurologist, the patient had fluctuating levels of consciousness with GCS scores that varied between 6 and 14, and patchy orientation to time and place. He had slight dysarthria and a skew deviation with hypertropia of the right eye.

Neurological scores: NIHSS 2, mRS 2, Barthel 95.

Special studies

Stroke MRI showed bithalamic acute infarcts without a vessel abnormality. In particular, the basilar artery had no persistent obstruction (Figure 13.1). Extensive testing for a possible source of embolism was negative, leading to the assumption of coronary angiography-associated stroke. For the course of the next two weeks, he showed gradual recovery of consciousness; however, he complained about drowsiness up to transfer to rehabilitation. Neuropsychological evaluation showed persisting disturbance of orientation in time and place with a mini-mental state examination (MMSE) score of 25 out of 30. He had impaired visuoconstructional skills, figurative memory, and attention.

More Case Studies in Stroke, eds. Michael G. Hennerici, Rolf Kern, Louis R. Caplan, and Kristina Szabo. Published by Cambridge University Press. © Cambridge University Press 2014.

Imaging findings

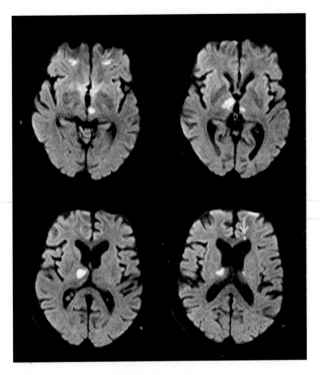

Figure 13.1. DWI shows bithalamic acute ischemic lesions in the territory of the right tuberothalamic artery and the left paramedian artery. An additional dot-like lesion is seen adjacent to the anterior horn of the lateral ventricle. The infarct pattern suggests a proximal source of embolism.

Diagnosis

Bithalamic infarcts.

General remarks

Bilateral thalamic infarcts is an uncommon pattern of acute stroke, typically located in the territories of the paramedian arteries when an unpaired paramedian artery arises from the P1 segment of the PCA and supplies both thalami. This pattern of ischemia was first dubbed top-of-the-basilar syndrome. In a study by Kumral and coworkers, patients with bithalamic infarction represented 0.6% of ischemic stroke patients. While previously it has been assumed to be a consequence of small vessel disease, more recent studies revealed an embolic cause in most patients. MRA can be used to demonstrate an underlying macroscopic vascular pathology of the basilar artery or the PCA, but the fine perforating thalamic arteries usually cannot be displayed by routine MRI at 1.5 or 3.0 Tesla due to their small diameter. In our case (as in 50% of the Kumral series), the lesions are located in two different vascular territories of the thalamus. This might be a mere coincidence in embolic stroke, or more likely be due to the individual vascular anatomy, as the patient had an absent P1 segment on the right and a hypoplastic P1 segment on the left side.

Special remarks

Paramedian thalamic infarctions produce a classical triad consisting of an acute decrease of arousal–especially in patients with bilateral lesions– neuropsychological abnormalities with a dysexecutive syndrome and with memory impairment and aphasia in left-sided lesions on occasion, and abnormal vertical gaze. Polar or tuberothalamic infarcts are characterized by neuropsychological symptoms with executive dysfunction, memory loss and altered arousal and orientation, impairments of learning and memory, and changes in personality. A specific clinical picture is reported to be found in up to 50% of the patients with bithalamic infarction. In bilateral paramedian infarction, this includes disorder of consciousness, memory dysfunctions, various types of vertical gaze palsy, and psychiatric changes. The alterations of consciousness are believed to be a result of a disruption of the extensive corticothalamic networks that regulate sleep and wakefulness. Interestingly, cognitive functions in patients with bilateral paramedian infarction have been described as not changing significantly over time, in contrast to those with infarcts in different arterial territories.

SUGGESTED READING

Caplan L. Top of the basilar syndrome: selected clinical aspects. *Neurology* 1980; **30**: 72–9.

Kumral E, Evyapan D, Balkir K, et al. Bilateral thalamic infarction. Clinical, etiological and MRI correlates. *Acta Neurol Scand* 2001; **103**: 35–42.

Roitberg BZ, Tuccar E, Alp MS. Bilateral paramedian thalamic infarct in the presence of an unpaired thalamic perforating artery. *Acta Neurochir* 2002; **144**: 301–4.

Schmahmann JD. Vascular syndromes of the thalamus. *Stroke* 2003; **34**: 2264–78.

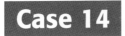

"I can still write"

Caroline Ottomeyer and Kristina Szabo

Clinical history

A 61-year-old right-handed dentist with treated hypertension awoke with acute loss of speech and saliva running out of the right corner of his mouth. He wrote "stroke" on a piece of paper for his wife, who called the ambulance.

Examination

In the emergency room, he was nearly mute due to grossly deficient motor output, but he had full comprehension of speech, and could communicate through gestures and intact, fluent writing; he wrote "I can still write" on a piece of paper. Speech was very difficult with strangled vowels, severe phonemic paraphasia, and abnormal prosody that was not facilitated by singing, reading, or repetition. This and the constant effort to correct himself accumulated in visible frustration, whereas, surprisingly, the patient was able to produce–apparently emotionally triggered–short but intact and fluently articulated commentaries of the situation (e.g., "It's not working!", "That's terrible!"). There was a slight right facial palsy without further affection of coordinated buccofacial movement (whistling, etc.) or oropharyngeal sensibility.

Neurological scores: NIHSS 4; Barthel 95; GCS 15.

Special studies

DWI performed shortly after presentation to the emergency room showed an acute ischemic lesion of the left precentral gyrus that was not yet visible on T2-weighted FLAIR images. The lesion extended medially slightly to the posterior part of the premotor cortex (Figure 14.1). Ultrasound and MRA showed a high-grade stenosis of the left ICA. As extensive stroke workup failed to show an alternative source of embolism, symptomatic ICA stenosis was considered the

More Case Studies in Stroke, eds. Michael G. Hennerici, Rolf Kern, Louis R. Caplan, and Kristina Szabo. Published by Cambridge University Press. © Cambridge University Press 2014.

most likely cause of stroke and the patient was treated with carotid endarterectomy on day 4.

Follow-up

Under logotherapy, the symptoms improved gradually and speech became more and more fluent after day 3. While in the beginning, due to the effort of speech, syntax was incomplete, but it was intact by day 3. At one week, the patient recovered completely including the right facial palsy.

Imaging findings

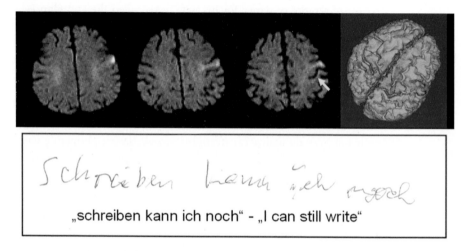

„schreiben kann ich noch" - „I can still write"

Figure 14.1. DWI shows a circumscribed hyperintense acute ischemic lesion in the left precentral gyrus (yellow arrows mark the central sulcus). On the far right: three-dimensional visualization of the lesion causing aphemia attained through segmentation, reformation, and registration of two-dimensional data sets (transparent brain tissue, ventricles in blue, lesion in red).

Diagnosis

Aphemia due to an ischemic lesion of the left precentral gyrus.

General remarks

Still not clearly classified as an articulatory or language disorder, aphemia is understood today as an isolated disorder of the planning of motor articulation of speech. These patients, even when mute, can write correctly and have no difficulty in the production of verbal sequences as long as they do not have to articulate them, distinguishing the disorder from motor aphasia. The presentation of abnormal prosody, "false starts," self corrections, and the occurrence of undisturbed "islands" in speech can help to differentiate it from dysarthria. Often, right-sided hemiparesis, limb apraxia, mild buccofacial apraxia, and central right facial palsy are associated symptoms.

Special remarks

The lesion of the precentral gyrus in this patient corresponds to recent information from a few similar published cases. These case studies link the control of articulation to a cortical region adjacent to the face motor cortex. Similarly, functional imaging studies have shown representational sites of tongue, lip, and articulation movements located in the pre- (M1) and postcentral (S1) gyrus without significant activation in Broca's and Wernicke's areas. Lesions of the premotor cortex, the insula, and Broca's area in the dominant hemisphere also have been observed causing aphemia-like syndromes. This widespread lesion pattern could suggest an underlying network involving the motor cortex, Broca's area, and supplementary motor areas engineering the articulation of speech.

FIRST DESCRIPTION

Broca P. Perte de la parole, ramollissement chronique et destruction partielle du lobe antérieur gauche du cerveau. *Bull Soc Anthrop* 1861; **2**: 235–8.

SUGGESTED READING

Hillis AE, Work M, Barker PB, et al. Re-examining the brain regions crucial for orchestrating speech articulation. *Brain* 2004; **127**: 1479–87.

Lotze M, Seggewies G, Erb M, Grodd W, Birbaumer N. The representation of articulation in the primary sensorimotor cortex. *Neuroreport* 2000; **11**: 2985–9.

Rheims S, Nighoghossian N, Hermier M, et al. Aphemia related to premotor cortex infarction. *Eur Neurol* 2006; **55**: 225–6.

Terao Y, Ugawa Y, Yamamoto T, et al. Primary face motor area as the motor representation of articulation. *J Neurol* 2007; **254**: 442–7.

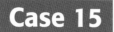

Old lady with sudden confusion

Kristina Szabo

Clinical history

A 74-year-old lady was admitted to the stroke unit due to the acute onset of a receptive aphasia that had started approximately 24 hours earlier. Within the first day, her symptoms resolved completely. She had a previously diagnosed atrial fibrillation, but was not taking an oral anticoagulant. She had had a left hemispheric stroke several years earlier. Initial MRI showed a chronic infarct in the left MCA territory and an acute ischemic stroke on DWI in a close vicinity.

On day 3, she developed sudden confusion with disorientation, stereotypical repetitive actions (e.g., searching for her purse), and amnesia. MRI was ordered, expecting recurrent left hemispheric stroke.

Examination

On neurological examination at admission the patient was awake and alert but had a fluent aphasia characterized by semantically inappropriate and paraphasic language and impaired language comprehension.

Neurological scores: NIHSS 4, Barthel 95, GCS 15.

Special studies

MRI on day 1 confirmed acute left MCA stroke in the left temporo-parietal region, involving the classic area of Wernicke with persistent vessel obstruction in the distal part of the left MCA. In addition, chronic left MCA stroke was seen on T2 images (Figure 15.1). Holter electroencephalography (EEG) on the stroke unit reaffirmed atrial fibrillation.

On MRI performed 72 hours later, a new hyperintense signal change on DWI was noted in the left hippocampus, associated with signs of hyperperfusion on time-to-peak maps in the PCA territory on PWI and MRA (Figure 15.2).

More Case Studies in Stroke, eds. Michael G. Hennerici, Rolf Kern, Louis R. Caplan, and Kristina Szabo. Published by Cambridge University Press. © Cambridge University Press 2014.

Imaging findings

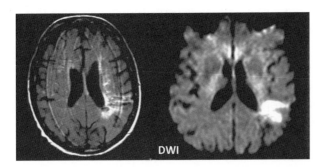

Figure 15.1. T2-weighted MRI at admission confirms reported left MCA stroke and shows an acute ischemic lesion in the left temporoparietal region, causing acute sensory aphasia.

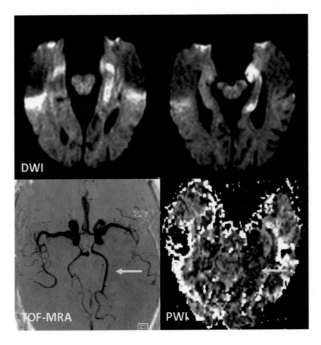

Figure 15.2. On MRI performed on day 3, a new hyperintense signal change on DWI is seen in the left hippocampus (upper row). This abnormality is accompanied by signs of hyperperfusion on MRA and on time-to-peak maps in the PCA territory on PWI (yellow arrows). Additional vascular pathology of the left MCA (red arrow) is present.

Diagnosis

Seizure-associated DWI abnormalities after left MCA stroke.

Follow-up

The left PCA territory showed focal hyperperfusion, indicating that ictal activity and not ischemia was responsible for the morphological changes in the hippocampus. EEG performed immediately after imaging confirmed complex partial status epilepticus with left temporal rhythmic sharp waves. The patient was treated with a benzodiazepine, after which her confusion resolved gradually. Since then, she has been hospitalized repeatedly due to symptomatic epilepsy, but has not had further strokes.

General remarks

The combination of (mostly transient) focal hyperintensity on DWI with corresponding hyperperfusion is an increasingly recognized phenomenon in the peri-ictal phase of (especially prolonged) epileptic seizures. These findings are hypothesized to be a consequence of transient metabolic and hemodynamic changes that are known to occur during seizure activity, leading to local, ictal-induced cytotoxic/vasogenic edema. The most common localization of DWI abnormalities associated with ictal activity is the hippocampus and the pulvinar of the thalamus. Both structures are known to play an important role in epileptogenesis and seizure propagation.

Special remarks

This case presents a challenging constellation of findings, but with a careful clinical examination and experience with ictal phenomena on MRI, it is possible to differentiate between ischemic and ictal/metabolic lesions. Keep in mind that hyperintense DWI signal change restricted to the hippocampus, accompanied by signs of hyperperfusion, may provide a diagnostic clue to the underlying ictal pathology of prolonged confusional syndromes, especially in the elderly or in patients with other primary CNS pathologies.

SUGGESTED READING

Chatzikonstantinou A, Gass A, Förster A, Hennerici MG, Szabo K. Features of acute DWI abnormalities related to status epilepticus. *Epilepsy Res* 2011; **97**: 45–51.

Chu K, Kang DW, Kim JY, Chang KH, Lee SK. Diffusion-weighted magnetic resonance imaging in nonconvulsive status epilepticus. *Arch Neurol* 2001; **58**: 993–8.

Kim JA, Chung JI, Yoon PH, et al. Transient MR signal changes in patients with generalized tonicoclonic seizure or status epilepticus: periictal diffusion-weighted imaging. *Am J Neuroradiol* 2001; **22**: 1149–60.

Szabo K, Poepel A, Pohlmann-Eden B, et al. Diffusion- and perfusion-weighted MRI demonstrates parenchymal changes in complex partial status epilepticus. *Brain* 2005; **128**: 1369–76.

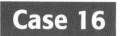

Case 16

Neck pain and upper arm paresis

Ralph Werner, Miriam M. Pfeiffer, Johannes C. Wöhrle

Clinical history

A 52-year-old man presented with a history of neck pain for nine days that became much worse after chiropractic therapy during the last six days. The head discomfort began to radiate to the left shoulder region. He had noticed a paresis of the upper arm for two days prior to admission.

Examination

On admission, clinical examination revealed paresis of C5 and C6 muscles of the left arm with the following Medical Research Council grades: upper arm abduction and elevation 2, upper arm external rotation 4−, elbow flexion 4. The deep tendon reflexes of the left biceps brachii and brachioradialis muscles were absent, while those of the left triceps brachii and all other muscles were normal. Only a small area of sensory impairment was found in the left lateral proximal upper arm. Coordination and cranial nerves were normal.

Neurological scores: NIHSS 4, mRS 3, GCS 15.

Special studies

Color-coded duplex sonography of the cervical arteries did not show signs of stenosis or oclusion; however, the vessel wall in the left V1-/V2-segment of the VA seemed thickened by echolucent material (Figure 16.1).

MRI showed a circular hematoma of the left VA in the V2 segment, compressing the nearby C5 and C6 nerve roots (Figure 16.2). MRA showed an irregular vessel lumen of the left VA due to dissection; MRI of the brain was completely normal.

More Case Studies in Stroke, eds. Michael G. Hennerici, Rolf Kern, Louis R. Caplan, and Kristina Szabo.
Published by Cambridge University Press. © Cambridge University Press 2014.

Follow-up

Antithrombotic medication with acetylsalicylic acid was initiated and physical therapy was started. The clinical evaluation after four weeks showed improved shoulder abduction and upper arm elevation to grade 3–4.

Imaging findings

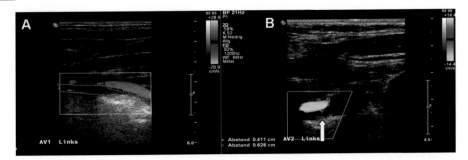

Figure 16.1. (A): duplex sonography of the left VA in the V1 segment. Echolucent material adjacent to the vessel wall, presumably due to a hematoma, is marked with a dotted line. (B): duplex sonography of the left VA, V2 segment. Arrow indicates hematoma in the vessel wall.

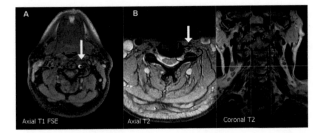

Figure 16.2. (A): typical "fried egg shape," semilunar vessel wall hematoma of the left VA with hyperintense signal in T1-weighted fat saturated transversal MRI (arrow). (B): vessel wall hematoma of the left VA in axial T2-weighted MRI (arrow); note the close proximity to the left fifth cervical root; the corresponding coronal T2-weighted MRI indicates the level of the axial image.

Diagnosis

Proximal vertebral artery dissection (VAD) with a wall hematoma-related compressive left C5/C6-radiculopathy.

General remarks

VAD is associated rarely with cervical compressive radiculopathy (1%–3%), and then also results in posterior circulation ischemia.

In the presence of neck pain, isolated arm paresis due to radiculopathy as the sole manifestation of VAD is exceedingly rare.

Special remarks

The diagnosis of VAD can be very difficult in cases of missing signs of cerebral ischemia and negative ultrasound findings of stenosis.

Radiculopathy as the only neurological manifestation of VAD may be confused easily with cervical disk prolapse, plexopathy of Parsonage–Turner syndrome, etc.

To diagnose VAD in this setting is important, as one would want to initiate antithrombotic therapy and avoid steroids for their thrombogenic potential.

CURRENT REVIEW

Arnold M, Kurmann R, Galimanis A, et al. Differences in demographic characteristics and risk factors in patients with spontaneous vertebral artery dissections with and without ischemic events. *Stroke* 2010; **41**: 802–4.

SUGGESTED READING

Arnold M, Bousser MG, Fahrni G, et al. Vertebral artery dissection: presenting findings and predictors of outcome. *Stroke* 2006; **37**: 2499–503.

Benny BV, Nagpal AS, Singh P, Smuck M. Vascular causes of radiculopathy: a literature review. *Spine J* 2011; **11**: 73–85.

Crum B, Mokri B, Fulgham J. Spinal manifestations of vertebral artery dissection. *Neurology* 2000; **55**: 304–6.

Dubard T, Pouchot J, Lamy C, et al. Upper limb peripheral deficits due to extracranial-vertebral artery dissection. *Cerebrovasc Dis* 1994; **4**: 88–91.

Hardmeier M, Haller S, Steck A, et al. Vertebral artery dissection presenting with fifth cervical root (C5) radiculopathy. *J Neurol* 2007; **254**: 672–3.

McGillion SF, Weston-Simons S, Harvey JR. Vertebral artery dissection presenting with multilevel combined sensorimotor radiculopathy: a case report and literature review. *J Spinal Disord Tech* 2009; **22**: 456–8.

Tabatabai G, Schöber W, Ernemann U, Weller M, Krüger R. Vertebral artery dissection presenting with ispilateral acute C5 and C6 sensorimotor radiculopathy: a case report. *Cases J* 2008; **1**: 139.

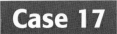
Aphasia during pregnancy

Ralph Werner and Johannes C. Wöhrle

Clinical history

A 35-year-old woman had a history of migraine with aura. She was in her 27th week of pregnancy when she presented with acute aphasia for one hour without headache. Cerebrovascular risk factors included hypercholesterolemia, former smoking, and a persistent foramen ovale.

Examination

Neurological examination showed a nonfluent, mixed aphasia with difficulties in verbal understanding and a slight right-sided brachiofacial hemiparesis. Deep tendon reflexes of arms and legs were symmetrically normal and Babinski's signs were negative. Sensation of light touch, pain, and vibration was unimpaired. Coordination of the right upper limb was impaired within the range of the paresis, while gait was normal.

Neurological scores: NIHSS 7, mRS 3, GCS 15.

Special studies

Immediate cerebral MRI of a stroke protocol showed a faint DWI hyperintensity with a corresponding attenuation on the ADC map in the anterior territory of the left MCA with normal appearance in the FLAIR sequence, indicating acute ischemic stroke (Figure 17.1A).

MRA supported the diagnosis of a high-grade M2 branch stenosis as suggested by transcranial color-coded duplex sonography (TCCS), with a flow velocity reduction of more than 30% in the left M1 segment as compared to the right MCA (Figure 17.2).

Extensive coagulation studies were normal including antiphospholipid antibodies but antinuclear antibody titers were elevated to 1:640.

More Case Studies in Stroke, eds. Michael G. Hennerici, Rolf Kern, Louis R. Caplan, and Kristina Szabo.
Published by Cambridge University Press. © Cambridge University Press 2014.

Follow-up

After informed consent from the husband, the patient received i.v. r-tPA at a dose of 0.9 mg/kg body weight over one hour, starting 1.75 h after onset of symptoms. The patient fully recovered within one hour after the end of i.v. r-tPA administration. Anticoagulation was started after 24 h with subcutaneous low molecular weight heparin (Dalteparin 5000 I.U. s.c. b.i.d.) for the rest of the pregnancy. At term, the patient delivered a healthy baby (2700 g, 47 cm, Apgar index 9-10-10).

Imaging findings

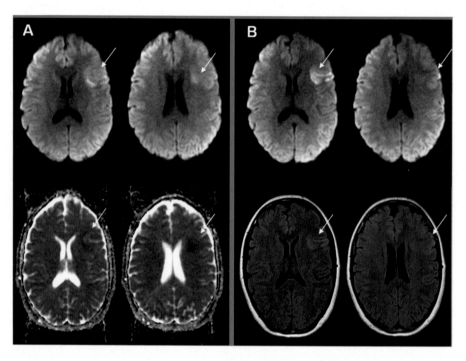

Figure 17.1. (A): MRI on admission showing a faint DWI hyperintensity with a corresponding ADC attenuation in the anterior territory of the left MCA (arrows). (B): MRI the day after thrombolysis still showing the restricted diffusion in DWI and a new hyperintensity in the FLAIR images, indicating the definite infarction that was smaller than the tissue at risk as seen on the ADC images before treatment (arrows).

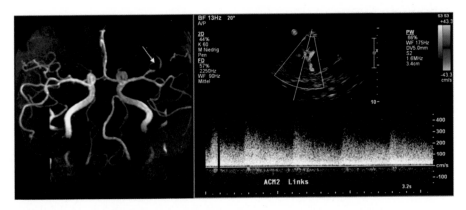

Figure 17.2. MRA and TCCS before thrombolysis displaying the high-grade stenosis of a frontal M2 branch of the left MCA (arrow).

Diagnosis

Embolic stroke with acute mixed aphasia and mild brachiofacial hemiparesis in pregnancy.

General remarks

Although cerebrovascular complications of pregnancy are well recognized, the data on i.v. r-tPA in acute ischemic stroke of pregnant women is exceedingly scarce.

Special remarks

The use of r-tPA in pregnant women is neither particularly tested nor recommended. In rabbits, but not in rats, r-tPA was embryotoxic at 3 mg/kg body weight; however, it is known not to cause fetal toxicity or teratogenicity but data are very limited; i.v. r-tPA does not cross the placenta. Case reports of i.v. r-tPA in pregnant women with stroke report diverse fetal outcomes with a range from healthy delivery to death. In a large summary of pregnant women receiving i.v. thrombolytic therapy for medical conditions other than stroke, the occurrence of preterm deliveries was between 6% and 8%.

On the basis of an individual judgment including ethical considerations of maternal and fetal risks, i.v. r-tPA may be considered in severe ischemic stroke in pregnant women.

CURRENT REVIEW

Li Y, Margraf J, Kluck B, Jenny D, Castaldo J. Thrombolytic therapy for ischemic stroke secondary to paradoxical embolism in pregnancy: a case report and literature review. *Neurologist* 2012; **18**: 44–8.

SUGGESTED READING

Allais G, Gabellari IC, Borgogno P, De Lorenzo C, Benedetto C. The risks of women with migraine during pregnancy. *Neurol Sci* 2010; **31**: S59–61.

Cronin CA, Weisman CJ, Llinas RH. Stroke treatment: beyond the three-hour window and in the pregnant patient. *Ann N Y Acad Sci* 2008; **1142**: 159–78.

Dapprich M, Boessenecker W. Fibrinolysis with alteplase in a pregnant woman with stroke. *Cerebrovasc Dis* 2002; **13**: 290.

De Keyser J, Gdovinová Z, Uyttenboogaart M, Vroomen PC, Luijckx GJ. Intravenous alteplase for stroke: beyond the guidelines and in particular. *Stroke* 2007; **38**: 2612–18.

Del Zotto E, Giossi A, Volonghi I, et al. Ischemic stroke during pregnancy and puerperium. *Stroke Res Treat* 2011 [Epub before print]

Sidorov EV, Feng W, Caplan LR. Stroke in pregnant and postpartum women. *Expert Rev Cardiovasc Ther* 2011; **9**: 1235–47.

Tate J, Bushnell C. Pregnancy and stroke risk in women. *Womens Health* 2011; **7**: 363–74.

Turrentine MA, Braems G, Ramirez MM. Use of thrombolytics for the treatment of thromboembolic disease during pregnancy. *Obstet Gynecol Surv* 1995; **50**: 534–41.

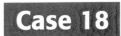

Case 18

Hemiparesis in two men treated for prostate carcinoma

James A. Adams

Clinical history: Patient 1

A 67-year-old man was admitted after the sudden onset of left hemiparesis three days following the sixth cycle of docetaxol chemotherapy. He had high-grade carcinoma of the prostate (Gleeson score 8) with bone metastases. Risk factors for cerebrovascular disease included hypertension, heavy alcohol intake, and pipe smoking.

Examination

Examination showed a severe left hemiparesis including the face, arm, and leg. He had hemisensory loss and visual inattention to the left. He had slight dysarthria.
Neurological scores: NIHSS 20, mRS 5.

Special studies

Brain CT showed low attenuation within the right cerebral cortex consistent with a subacute ischemic stroke (Figure 18.1). Doppler examination revealed no significant atherosclerotic disease of the carotid circulation. His ECG was normal. A 24-hour Holter monitor showed no atrial fibrillation. TEE showed preserved biventricular function with no evidence of mural thrombus or myxoma.

Follow-up

He received stroke unit management with nasogastric feeding, antiplatelets, and multidisciplinary therapy. Following a protracted admission with several hospital-acquired infections, he died from an acute pancreatitis of unknown etiology.

More Case Studies in Stroke, eds. Michael G. Hennerici, Rolf Kern, Louis R. Caplan, and Kristina Szabo. Published by Cambridge University Press. © Cambridge University Press 2014.

Imaging findings

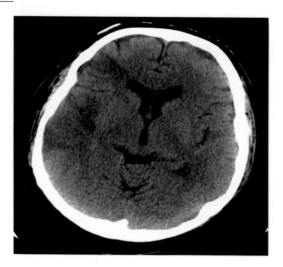

Figure 18.1. Cross-sectional CT of the brain demonstrates low attenuation and loss of gray/white matter differentiation in the right MCA territory consistent with subacute ischemic stroke.

Diagnosis

He was diagnosed with a cryptogenic right MCA ischemic stroke. It was postulated that the etiology of his stroke was an idiosyncratic drug reaction following the administration of docetaxol chemotherapy, combined with a susceptibility for thromboembolic complications relating to his underlying malignancy.

Clinical history: Patient 2

A 74-year-old man was admitted with sudden-onset left hemiparesis three weeks following the fourth cycle of docetaxol chemotherapy. He had advanced carcinoma of the prostate with metastases to bone and local pelvic infiltration. His only risk factor for ischemic stroke was hypertension.

Examination

Examination revealed a minor left hemiparesis of the face, arm, and leg. He had no speech, sensory, or visual field deficits.

Neurological scores: NIHSS 5, mRS 3.

Special studies

DWI of the brain revealed areas of restricted diffusion in the posterior limb of the right internal capsule, the right medial temporal lobe, and the left occipital lobe (Figure 18.2). MRA of the extracranial vessels revealed no significant extracranial atherosclerotic disease in the anterior or posterior circulations. His ECG was normal and a seven-day loop recording of the heart revealed no atrial fibrillation. Contrast-enhanced transthoracic "bubble" echocardiography was unremarkable and did not reveal a significant ASD.

Follow-up

He received hyperacute stroke unit care including antiplatelet therapy with aspirin and risk factor modification. He developed acute bilateral pulmonary emboli shortly after the acute stroke and had an inferior vena cava filter inserted to prevent further thromboembolic complications. He was fully anticoagulated with warfarin at two weeks poststroke. All neurological deficits resolved with after-therapy and he was discharged three weeks poststroke.

Imaging findings

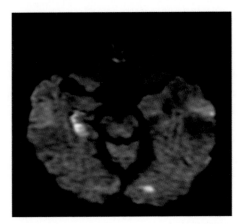

Figure 18.2. DWI of the brain reveals restricted diffusion in the right internal capsule (not shown), the right medial temporal lobe, and left occipital lobe consistent with acute ischemic stroke.

Diagnosis

Cryptogenic bihemispheric ischemic strokes (right temporal lobe, right posterior limb of the internal capsule, and left occipital lobe). Given that the event occurred three weeks after treatment with docetaxol, we posited that his stroke may have been precipitated by the effects of drug metabolites on normal hemostasis in conjunction with a hypercoagulable state induced by his underlying carcinoma.

General remarks

The incidence of stroke in patients with cancer is unknown–14.6% of patients with solid extracranial tumors were found to have pathological evidence of cerebrovascular disease at postmortem; however, only 7.4% had been symptomatic with strokes. Several factors make cancer patients more prone to developing ischemic stroke (Table 18.1). This association is poorly understood but it is well recognized that cancer induces a hypercoagulable state disrupting normal clotting physiology and making thromboembolic disease more likely in susceptible individuals. Tumors may induce cardioembolic strokes through direct tumor embolization (e.g., atrial myxoma) or associated inflammatory disease (marantic or non-bacterial endocarditis). There may be direct compression of extra- or intracranial arteries from primary or metastatic cancer. Several antineoplastic therapies have been implicated in the etiology of strokes in cancer patients. It is well established that radiotherapy to the neck can accelerate extracranial atherosclerotic stenosis, predisposing to stroke.

Special remarks

Ischemic stroke is recognized as a rare complication of antineoplastic therapy. Retrospective data estimates the incidence of stroke among oncology patients receiving chemotherapy to be 0.415%. The largest study looked at 10 963 cancer

Table 18.1. Causes of ischemic stroke in cancer patients

Hypercoagulable state
Non-bacterial (marantic) endocarditis
Tumor embolism (including atrial myxoma)
Radiotherapy-induced vasculopathy
Surgery
Chemotherapy
Direct compression of intracranial or extracranial arteries
Opportunistic infection

Table 18.2. Postulated mechanisms of chemotherapy-induced stroke

Idiosyncratic reaction
Induction of a hypercoagulable state
Increased von Willebrand factor levels
Reduced protein C concentration
Activation of platelets
Influx of circulatory mucin from tumor lysis
Endothelial injury from free radical toxicity
Vasospasm from hypomagnesemia

patients in Taiwan. Embolic MCA infarction was the most common stroke syndrome. Sixty percent of strokes occurred after the first cycle of treatment. As with patient 1, nearly 75% of strokes occurred within 10 days of administration of the chemotherapy. This was posited to be a direct effect of the drug whereas strokes occurring several weeks following administration, as in patient 2, were postulated to be a result of drug metabolites. Currently there is very limited prospective data available with two papers reporting just one stroke out of 288 patients (0.347%).

Platinum-containing chemotherapies, in particular cisplatin, have been implicated in the etiology of ischemic strokes in many case reports and this is the most common agent found in retrospective reviews. Despite this being the most extensively studied drug, the exact mechanisms by which it induces thromboembolic disease remain unknown. Postulated mechanisms of chemotherapy-induced stroke are highlighted in Table 18.2. These include the induction of a hypercoagulable state by increased von Willebrand factor levels, a reduction in protein C concentration, activation of platelets, and an influx of circulatory mucin from tumor lysis. In addition, cisplatin may induce vascular endothelial injury via direct free radical toxicity and vasospasm caused by hypomagnesemia.

Docetaxol is a Taxane chemotherapy isolated from the bark of the Pacific yew tree, which acts to hyperstabilize microtubules, thus inhibiting mitosis. To our knowledge, no cases of docetaxol-associated ischemic stroke in patients with prostate cancer have been reported, and there is no data to explain possible mechanisms of docetaxol-induced vascular injury. How we identify and monitor vulnerable cancer patients and minimize the risk of them developing stroke sequelae remains an important research and clinical question.

CURRENT REVIEW

Grisold W, Oberndorfer S, Struhal W. Stroke and cancer: a review. *Acta Neurol Scand* 2009; **119**: 1–16.

SUGGESTED READING

Amico L, Caplan LR, Thomas C. Cerebrovascular complications of mucinous cancers. *Neurology* 1989; **39**: 522–6.

Cestari DM, Weine DM, Panageas KS, Segal AZ, DeAngelis LM. Stroke in patients with cancer. *Neurology* 2004; **62**: 2025–30.

Cheng SW, Wu LL, Ting AC, et al. Irradiation induced extracranial carotid stenosis in patients with head and neck malignancies. *Am J Surg* 1999; **178**: 323–8.

Graus F, Rogers LR, Posner JB. Cerebrovascular complications in patients with cancer. *Medicine* 1985; **64**: 16–35.

Grisold W, Oberndorfer S, Struhal W. Stroke and cancer: a review. *Acta Neurol Scand* 2009; **119**: 1–16.

Li SH, Chen WH, Tang Y, et al. Incidence of ischaemic stroke post-chemotherapy: a retrospective review of 10,963 patients. *Clin Neurol Neurosurg* 2006; **108**(2): 150–6.

Nichols CR, Roth JB, Williams SD, et al. No evidence of acute cardiovascular complications of chemotherapy for testicular cancer: an analysis of the Testicular Cancer Intergroup Study. *J Clin Oncol* 1992; **10**(5): 760–5.

Numico G, Garrone O, Dongiovanni V, et al. Prospective evaluation of major vascular events in patients with non-small cell lung carcinoma treated with cisplatin and gemcitabine. *Cancer* 2005; **103**(5): 994–9.

Rogers LR. Cerebrovascular complications in cancer patients. *Neurol Clin N Am* 2003; **21**: 167–92.

Schwazbach CJ, Schaefer A, Ebert A, et al. Stroke and cancer: the importance of cancer-associated hypercoagulation as a possible stroke etiology. *Stroke* 2012; **43**(11): 3029–34.

Horner syndrome and headache

Paolo Costa and Alessandro Pezzini

Clinical history

A 39-year-old man with a history of arterial hypertension presented with a right-sided headache and a right Horner syndrome. Brain MRI and MRA investigations revealed no parenchymal lesion but a dissection of the right ICA (Figure 19.1A). No major or minor traumatic event was detectable in the patient's recent history. Intravenous unfractionated heparin was initiated followed by oral anticoagulation treatment, targeting an INR between 2 and 3. Four months later, the patient presented with an acute cerebral infarct in the territory of the left MCA. MRA showed a new dissection involving the left ICA (Figure 19.1B,C).

Examination

Neurological examination revealed Horner syndrome on the right side (as a consequence of the first ICA dissection), aphasia, and right hemiparesis with sensory loss. A physical examination revealed micrognathia, proptosis, absent lingual frenulum, pectuscarinatum, velvety skin, and dystrophic scars on both knees. A history of recurrent wrist dislocation was reported as well.

Neurological scores: NIHSS 8, mRS 3, GCS 15.

Special studies

Because of the evidence of clinical signs consistent with the hypothesis of connective tissue disorder, we performed sequence analyses of collagen type III, alpha 1 (COL3A1), transforming growth factor beta-receptors 1 (TGFBR1), small mother against decapentaplegic 3 (SMAD3), smooth muscle aortic alpha-actin (ACTA2), and fibrillin 1 (FBN1), which turned out to be negative. In contrast, sequence analysis of the *TGFBR2* gene revealed the novel c.1115A>G transition in exon 4, leading to the substitution p.K372R in the kinase domain of the receptor

More Case Studies in Stroke, eds. Michael G. Hennerici, Rolf Kern, Louis R. Caplan, and Kristina Szabo. Published by Cambridge University Press. © Cambridge University Press 2014.

(Figure 19.1D,E). Segregation analysis found the same *TGFBR2* mutation in the unaffected mother and one daughter (Figure 19.1F), in spite of the patient's unremarkable family history. These findings suggest incomplete penetrance of the mutation, as in the case of other *TGFBR* mutations.

Imaging findings

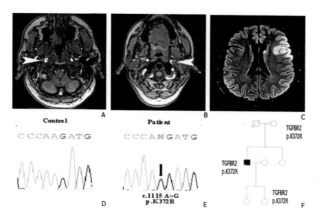

Figure 19.1. (A): first MRA (TE, 3D-TOF) showing right ICA dissection (white arrowhead). (B): second MRA (TE, 3D-TOF) showing left ICA dissection (white arrowhead). (C): MRI (T2-weighted) scan showing left MCA infarct. (D): *TGFBR2* sequencing in the index patient (E) and control individuals (D). (F): patient pedigree, black symbol, index patient.

Diagnosis

Recurrent ICA dissection caused by mutation in *TGFBR2*.

General remarks

Mutations in *TGFBR1* and *TGFBR2* have been associated recently with a widespread vascular involvement of complex phenotype, as a consequence of a defect in elastogenesis with loss of elastin content and disarray of the elastic fibers [1,2]. This may result in altered structure and composition of vascular extracellular matrix, predisposing to arterial dissection. All these findings are, actually, in line with the ultrastructural abnormalities observed in the skin and vessel wall of patients with spontaneous cervical artery dissection (sCAD) [3,4]. Therefore, the hypothesis that *TGFBR* mutations may cause sCAD is plausible.

In the present patient, we detected the novel p.K327R substitution affecting the kinase domain of TGFBR2, involved in TGF-β binding and signaling. Several arguments support the possible disease-causing effect of this mutation: (1) it was not detected in 500 chromosomes of control Italian blood donors; (2) it substitutes a highly conserved residue in the orthologs of the receptor; (3) it is predicted to influence protein function with high probability by PolyPhen tool bioinformatic analysis; the p.K372R missense mutation affects a residue in the TGFBR2 kinase domain like the majority of Loeys–Dietz syndrome mutations that have been identified to date.

This supports the hypothesis of involvement of TGF-β in sCAD-specific pathways and prompts speculation on disease pathogenesis. sCAD may be the phenotypic expression of a systemic inherited disorder of the extracellular matrix, even in sporadic cases with no major signs of connective tissue anomalies. Actually, our patient showed only mild signs of connective tissue involvement. As in cases of familiar thoracic aortic aneurysms and dissections (TAAD), in which the involvement of the aorta is the only clinical feature [5], a distinct clinical entity due to *TGFBR2* mutations with a presentation limited to cervical arteries cannot be excluded. Whether additional environmental or genetic factors influence the individual propensity to sCAD occurrence in *TGFBR2* mutation carriers remains to be determined.

Special remarks

Although mutations in *TGFBR2* are probably an infrequent cause of sCAD, the identification of subjects carrying the defective gene may have clinical implications for the individual and familial counseling. What remains unclear is how to identify sCAD patients who are more likely to carry the defective gene. As opposed to the familial clustering of dissection involving the thoracic aorta, familial aggregation is a rare finding in sCAD. The incomplete penetrance, the wide intrafamilial variability of *TGFBR2* mutations-related phenotypes, and the lack of genotype–phenotype correlations [6], make the picture even more confused. Thus, awaiting the results from larger series, the molecular characterization of *TGFBR* should be considered in all patients with sCAD, regardless of the presence of clinical features suggestive of connective tissue abnormalities.

REFERENCES

1. Loeys BL, Chen J, Neptune ER, et al. A syndrome of altered cardiovascular, craniofacial, neurocognitive and skeletal development caused by mutations in TGFBR1 or TGFBR2. *Nat Genet* 2005; **37**(3): 275–81.

2. Singh KK, Rommel K, Mishra A, et al. TGFBR1 and TGFBR2 mutations in patients with features of Marfan syndrome and Loeys-Dietz syndrome. *Hum Mutat* 2006; **27**(8): 770–7.

3. Brandt T, Orberk E, Weber R, et al. Pathogenesis of cervical artery dissections. Association with connective tissue abnormalities. *Neurology* 2001; **57**: 24–30.

4. Völker W, Besselmann M, Dittrich R, et al. Generalized arteriopathy in patients with cervical artery dissection. *Neurology* 2005; **64**: 1508–13.

5. Pannu H, Tran-Fadulu V, Milewicz DM. Genetic basis of thoracic aortic aneurysms and aortic dissections. *Am J Med Genet C Semin Med Genet* 2005; **139C**: 10–16.

6. Loeys BL, Schwarze U, Holm T, et al. Aneurysm syndromes caused by mutations in the TGF-beta receptor. *N Engl J Med* 2006; **355**(8): 788–98.

CURRENT REVIEW

Debette S, Leys D. Cervical-artery dissections: predisposing factors, diagnosis, and outcome. *Lancet Neurol* 2009; **8**(7): 668–78.

SUGGESTED READING

Drera B, Tadini G, Barlati S, Colombi M. Identification of a novel TGFBR1 mutation in a Loeys–Dietz syndrome type II patient with vascular Ehlers–Danlos syndrome phenotype. *Clin Genet* 2008; **73**: 290–3.

Pezzini A, Del Zotto E, Giossi A, et al. Transforming growth factor β signaling perturbation in the Loeys-Dietz syndrome. *Curr Med Chem* 2012; **19**(3): 454–60.

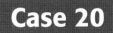

Involuntary shaking of the arm and leg

Sefanja Achterberg, Suzanne Persoon, L. Jaap Kappelle

Clinical history

A 56-year-old man presented with a short episode of language problems followed by recurrent short-lasting attacks of a shaking right arm and leg with loss of sensation. These attacks occurred four to five times a day and had a sudden onset (no march) of symptoms. Most attacks occurred soon after rising from a chair or walking a few steps. Ten years ago, he had transient episodes of dysarthric speech problems and a significant right carotid stenosis was found and he underwent carotid endarterectomy. A further medical history revealed an aortic aneurysm for which a bifurcation graft was placed, rheumatoid arthritis, hypertension, and hypercholesterolemia.

Examination

Neurological examination revealed no focal deficits. His blood pressure was 145/85 mmHg in the supine position and 135/90 mmHg after two minutes in the upright position. The carotid artery pulse was present on the right and absent on the left side, and no murmurs were heard.

Neurological scores: NIHSS 0, mRS 1.

Special studies

MRI FLAIR images showed signs of recent infarction in the left hemisphere, primarily in the caudate nucleus. MRA showed an occlusion of the left ICA. Conventional angiography showed a severe stenosis of the external and common left carotid artery, through which collateral blood flow to the left hemisphere came from the left ophthalmic artery. On the right side, the known carotid endarterectomy status was found, but additionally, a stenosis in the distal common carotid artery as well as an occlusion of the external carotid artery were seen (Figure 20.1).

More Case Studies in Stroke, eds. Michael G. Hennerici, Rolf Kern, Louis R. Caplan, and Kristina Szabo. Published by Cambridge University Press. © Cambridge University Press 2014.

Imaging findings

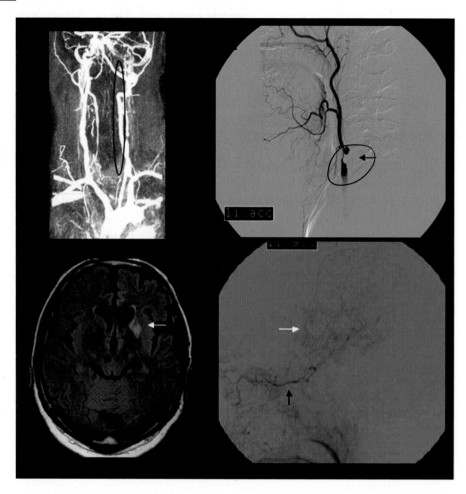

Figure 20.1. Left side: MRA showing occlusion of the left ICA (top row); FLAIR imaging showing infarction of the caudate nucleus in the left hemisphere (bottom row). Right side: Catheter angiography showing severe stenosis of the left common carotid artery (top row); filling of the ophthalmic artery with slightly visible intracranial blood flow through this artery and some leptomeningeal collaterals (bottom row).

Diagnosis

Limb-shaking TIAs.

General remarks

Shaking attacks of limbs are mostly diagnosed as epilepsy, but can also be a sign of compromised cerebral blood flow. Differentiation between these two diagnoses can be difficult but certain clues can be found with careful history taking. The mode of onset of symptoms may help their differentiation. Limb-shaking TIAs occur suddenly without a march of symptoms and are short lasting (mostly <5 min). There is no change of consciousness and usually there is accompanying paresis of the involved limb. Often, but not necessarily, TIAs may be precipitated by activities that compromise cerebral perfusion such as rising, exercise, or coughing.

Special remarks

There is no standardized treatment regime for patients with limb-shaking TIAs associated with an ICA occlusion. Since the attacks are thought to have a hemo-dynamic origin, a first treatment option might be the lowering or discontinuation of blood pressure-lowering medication, with the aim to increase the flow state of the brain. Other more invasive options are revascularization of an additional stenosis in the cerebropetal arteries, or extracranial-intracranial bypass surgery.

Initially, our patient had a carotid endarterectomy of the left common and external carotid arteries without effect on the frequency of the limb-shaking TIAs. Subsequently, we decided to perform a right-sided carotid endarterectomy to improve flow to the left hemisphere via the anterior communicating artery. After this second procedure, the limb-shaking TIAs did not occur.

SUGGESTED READING

Baquis GD, Pessin MS, Scott RM. Limb shaking–a carotid TIA. *Stroke* 1985; **16**(3): 444–8.
Persoon S, Kappelle LJ, Klijn CJ. Limb-shaking transient ischaemic attacks in patients with internal carotid artery occlusion: a case-control study. *Brain* 2010; **133**(3): 915–22.

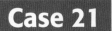

Case 21

A young woman with infertility

Patricia Martínez-Sánchez, Blanca Fuentes,
Exuperio Díez-Tejedor

Clinical history

A 33-year-old woman with a medical history of infertility and sudden loss of hearing one month earlier came to the emergency room because of acute speech difficulty and weakness involving the right face and arm. She had no history of cardiovascular risk factors.

Examination

On examination, she had motor aphasia, right faciobrachial hypesthesia, and motor weakness.

Neurological scores: NIHSS 10, mRS 4.

Special studies

The cerebral CT and ECG were normal. Carotid duplex showed a free-floating thrombus in the left ICA (Figure 21.1A,B) that was not producing flow acceleration. Arteriography was performed urgently to study the arterial patency and to remove the carotid thrombus. However, the thrombus had disappeared spontaneously without any clinical deterioration. A second carotid duplex and a carotid CTA two days later confirmed these results (Figure 21.1C). MRI showed infarction in the left MCA territory (Figure 21.2A). Peripheral blood showed a platelet count of 505×10^9/L. The JAK2V617F mutation was detected in peripheral blood samples by a multiple allele-specific polymerase chain reaction. Bone marrow aspiration showed clustered hyperlobulated megakaryocytes (Figure 21.2B,C). Additional studies, including an extensive battery of tests for coagulopathies and a complete cardiology study, were negative.

JAK 2

More Case Studies in Stroke, eds. Michael G. Hennerici, Rolf Kern, Louis R. Caplan, and Kristina Szabo.
Published by Cambridge University Press. © Cambridge University Press 2014.

Follow-up

Antiplatelet treatment was initiated as secondary stroke prevention. The patient had a good outcome, with progressive neurological improvement. Her three-month mRS was 1. The thrombocytosis decreased spontaneously, with a platelet count of 452×10^{10}/L after six months.

Imaging findings

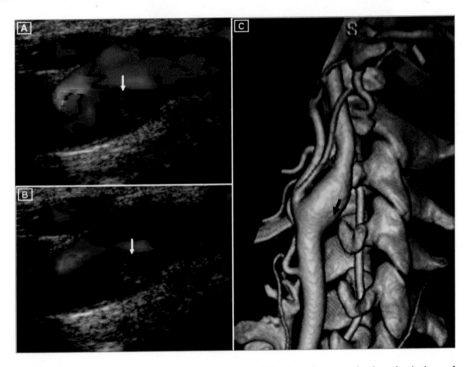

Figure 21.1. (A, B): carotid duplex with B-mode showing a mobile thrombus attached to the intima of the distal wall of the left ICA (arrow) during systole (A) and diastole (B). The intima–media thickness is increased at this point. (C): left ICA CTA demonstrates the absence of thrombi (arrow).

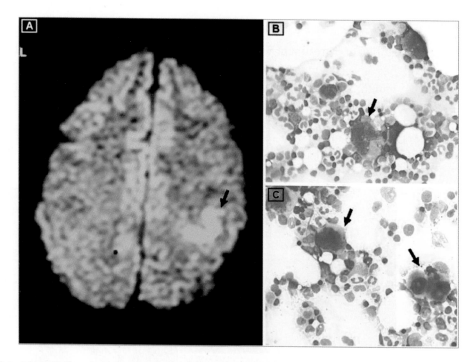

Figure 21.2. (A): DWI showing infarction in the left MCA territory (arrow). (B, C): Bone marrow aspirate showing clustered hyperlobulated megakaryocytes (arrows).

Diagnosis

The patient was diagnosed with stroke of unusual cause and essential thrombocythemia associated with the *JAK2V617F* mutation.

General remarks

The presence of a mobile, free-floating thrombus in the ICA as a cause of brain ischemia is infrequent and its natural history is not well understood. Some pathologies, such as thrombophilias, carotid dissections, trauma, and plaques, are associated with carotid thrombus, although in many cases the etiology is not identified. Myeloproliferative disorders, especially essential thrombocythemia and polycythemia vera, may be associated with thrombi development, mainly in veins. The risk of arterial thrombosis is increased significantly if patients have the *JAK2V617F* mutation (OR 2.49, 95% CI: 1.71–3.61), which has been found in approximately 50% of those individuals with essential thrombocythemia.

The pathophysiology of thrombosis in patients with essential thrombocythemia is complex. Traditionally, abnormalities of platelet number and function have been assumed to be the main players, but increased dynamic interactions between platelets, leukocytes, and the endothelium probably represent a fundamental interplay in generating a thrombophilic state. In addition, endothelial dysfunction, a well-known risk factor for vascular disease, may play a role in the thrombotic risk for patients with this disease. Recent studies reported that *JAK2V617F* carriers showed elevated expression levels of some procoagulant, adhesive, and inflammatory molecules by platelets and neutrophils compared to wild-type subjects. However, the presence of mobile floating thrombi in the extracranial carotid arteries associated with the presence of the *JAK2V617F* mutation is exceptional, especially in the presence of mild thrombocytosis, as in this case.

Special remarks

The presence of a free-floating thrombus in the ICA is rare, especially in young people without atherosclerosis. In these patients, uncommon causes of stroke such as cancer, especially adenocarcinomas, and inherited or acquired thrombophilias should be ruled out. Essential thrombocythemia, especially associated with the *JAK2* mutation, should be considered even in the case of mild thrombocytosis, after excluding secondary causes of thrombocythemia.

CURRENT REVIEW

Vianello F, Battisti A, Cella G, Marchetti M, Falanga A. Defining the thrombotic risk in patients with myeloproliferative neoplasms. *ScientificWorldJournal* 2011; **11**: 1131–7.

SUGGESTED READING

Bhatti AF, Leon LR Jr, Labropoulos N, et al. Free-floating thrombus of the carotid artery: literature review and case reports. *J Vasc Surg* 2007; **45**(1): 199–205.

Caplan L, Stein R, Patel D, et al. Intraluminal clot of the carotid artery detected angiographically. *Neurology* 1984; **34**: 1175–81.

Hill SL, Brozyna W. Extensive mobile thrombus of the internal carotid artery: a case report, treatment options, and review of the literature. *Am Surg* 2005; **71**: 853–5.

James C, Ugo V, Le Couedic JP, et al. A unique clonal JAK2 mutation leading to constitutive signalling causes polycythaemia vera. *Nature* 2005; **434**: 1144–8.

Larsen TS, Pallisgaard N, Møller MB, et al. High prevalence of arterial thrombosis in JAK2 mutated essential thrombocythaemia: independence of the V617F allele burden. *Hematology* 2008; **13**: 71–6.

Moreno MJ, Lozano ML, Roldán V, et al. JAK2V617F, hemostatic polymorphism, and clinical features as risk factors for arterial thombotic events in essential thrombocythemia. *Ann Hematol* 2008; **87**: 763–5.

Richard S, Perrin, J, Baillot PA, Lacour JC, Ducrocq X. Ischaemic stroke and essential thrombocytemia: a series of 14 cases. *Eur J Neurol* 2011; **18**: 995–8.

Tefferi A, Vardiman JW. Classification and diagnosis of myeloproliferative neoplasm: the 2008 World Health Organization criteria and point-of-care diagnostic algorithms. *Leukemia* 2008; **22**: 14–22.

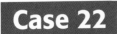

Acute weakness of the right lower limb

Angelika Alonso

Clinical fistory

A 65-year-old woman presented with the acute onset of weakness of the right lower limb. She had a prominent foot drop, and reported reduced sensibility to touch on the lateral ankle. The palsy was painless. She also denied back pain before the onset of leg weakness.

Examination

Neurological examination showed a peroneal-like distribution of right lower limb monoparesis, which predominantly affected ankle dorsiflection but spared knee and hip function. Sensory loss was limited to the lateral malleolus. The ipsilateral upper extremities and the face were not affected. Monosynaptic reflexes including the triceps surae reflex were equal bilaterally; Babinski's sign was negative.

Neurological scores: NIHSS 2, mRS 3, Barthel 75.

Special studies

On DWI, a small cortical infarction involving the contralateral superior and medial margin of the precentral gyrus was identified (Figure 22.1). MRA showed an occlusion of a distal branch of the right ACA, representing the paracentral lobule artery.

Motor neurography of the peroneal nerve was equal bilaterally and normal. Motor evoked potentials (EPs) showed no affection of the corticospinal tract.

Extra- and intracranial Doppler-/duplex sonography revealed slight atherosclerosis, but no relevant arterial stenosis or vessel occlusion. Holter ECG monitoring found no episodes of atrial fibrillation. TEE detected a PFO °III without concomitant atrial septal aneurysm as a potential source of cardiac embolism.

More Case Studies in Stroke, eds. Michael G. Hennerici, Rolf Kern, Louis R. Caplan, and Kristina Szabo. Published by Cambridge University Press. © Cambridge University Press 2014.

Imaging findings

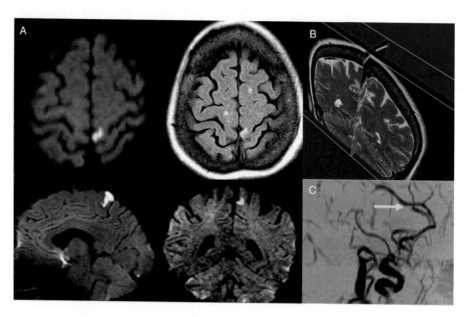

Figure 22.1. On DWI, a small cortical infarction involving the contralateral superior and medial margin of the precentral gyrus was identified (A). Through segmentation, reformation, and registration of two-dimensional data sets, a three-dimensional visualization of the ischemic lesion was computed (B). MRA demonstrated an occlusion of a distal branch of the right anterior cerebral artery, representing the paracentral lobule artery (C).

Diagnosis

Acute ischemic cortical infarction of the medial and superior margin of the precentral gyrus (ACA territory).

General remarks

Acute distal leg paresis, especially when presenting as foot drop, is suspected mainly to evolve from a peripheral nerve palsy. Leg-predominant weakness and monoparesis of the lower limb due to stroke have been described following hemispheric infarctions in the ACA or MCA territory, or along the course of the corticospinal tract and in the thalamus. However, small cortical lesions in the contralateral paracentral lobe on the medial and superior margin of the precentral gyrus can mimic a peripheral origin. Topographically, the lesions project over the foot motor area of the primary motor cortex. Owing to the small lesion size, the initial palsy grades are rather moderate, and complete to near-to-complete recovery is frequent. As a great portion of the primary motor cortex is still intact, motor EPs fail to detect an affection of the corticospinal tract.

Special remarks

Similarly to central distal lower limb paresis, cortical lesion patterns mimicking radial- or ulnar-like distributed palsies of the distal upper extremity have been reported. In these cases, cortical emboli involving the motor hand cortex attributable to distal Rolandic artery obstruction have been detected. Comparable to lower limb palsy, the observed clinical course mostly is benign.

SUGGESTED READING

Alonso A, Gass A, Griebe M, et al. Isolated ischaemic lesions in the foot motor area mimic peripheral lower-limb palsy. *J Neurol Neurosurg Psychiatry* 2010; **81**(7): 822–3.

Brust JCM. Anterior cerebral artery. In Caplan LR, van Gijn J (eds.), *Stroke Syndromes*, 3rd edn. Cambridge: Cambridge University Press, 2012; 364–74.

Gass A, Szabo K, Behrens S, Rossmanith C, Hennerici MG. A diffusion-weighted MRI study of acute ischemic distal arm paresis. *Neurology* 2001; **57**: 1589–94.

Schneider R, Gautier JC. Leg weakness due to stroke. Site of lesions, weakness patterns and causes. *Brain* 1994; **117**(2): 347–54.

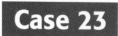

Recurrent embolic stroke in a 61-year-old man

Christopher Schwarzbach

Clinical history

A 61-year-old man presented with an acute left hemiparesis and speech arrest. He was first admitted to hospital only three months before this admission when he presented with acute bihemispheric infarction of presumably embolic origin. However, so far extensive diagnostic evaluation remained unrevealing and stroke etiology was not identified. At the time of this admission, the patient was given platelet inhibitors–a combination of aspirin and dipyridamole.

Examination

At admission, the patient had severe global aphasia and left hemiparesis. Previously, he had recovered well from his first stroke with moderate residual aphasia.
Neurological scores: NIHSS 10, Barthel 45, GCS 15.

Special studies performed during his admission for the first stroke

Extracranial Doppler/duplex sonography, MRA, and TEE were normal. Repeated ECG monitoring showed no evidence of atrial fibrillation or other cardiac arrhythmias. Transcranial ultrasound monitoring for high-intensity transient signals (HITS) and Bubbles were negative. Coagulation studies showed no abnormalities except for an elevation of D-dimer levels (3.3 µg/ml) without evidence of DVT.

Current studies

CTA of the aortic arch showed no aortic arch plaques. As a secondary finding, two solid round lesions of unknown degree of malignancy could be identified (Figure 23.1). A PET–CT additionally revealed metastasis in the mediastinum.

More Case Studies in Stroke, eds. Michael G. Hennerici, Rolf Kern, Louis R. Caplan, and Kristina Szabo. Published by Cambridge University Press. © Cambridge University Press 2014.

Biopsy verified an adenocarcinoma of the lung. D-dimer levels remained elevated (4.1 µg/ml).

Imaging findings

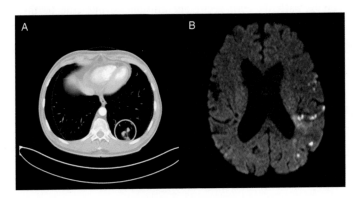

Figure 23.1. (A): CT of the chest showing a newly diagnosed pulmonary tumor. (B): DWI in the axial plane showing embolic scattering of infarction.

Diagnosis

Recurrent brain infarcts due to cancer-associated hypercoagulability.

General remarks

New data support the concept of cancer-associated hypercoagulability as a still widely underestimated, important risk factor for ischemic stroke in cancer patients. Additionally, other direct or indirect tumor-related conditions such as tumor embolism, vessel infiltration, or compression may contribute to the large range of cancer-associated causes of stroke. Ischemic stroke may precede the diagnosis of malignancy in a significant number of patients (up to a quarter of all ischemic stroke patients with concomitant malignant disease). Adenocarcinomas are associated with an elevated risk of ischemic stroke, namely lung- and pancreatic- but probably also gastric- and gastrointestinal cancers in general.

Special remarks

Evidence of small scattered brain infarcts, especially in the absence of other conventional stroke mechanisms, and strongly elevated D-dimer levels as a result of activation of the coagulation cascade are the most suggestive findings. Diagnostic evaluation in stroke patients with concomitant malignancy should include a broad laboratory assessment of hypercoagulability, including D-dimer levels and screening for other thromboembolic complications such as DVT. Non-bacterial thrombotic endocarditis (NBTE) may be a direct consequence of the disease as well. However, NBTE is hard to detect in the living patient, and therefore a rare finding even in patients with recurrent embolic stroke due to the coagulation disorder. Data concerning secondary prevention in this group of patients are still insufficient but beside tumor therapy, especially low molecular weight heparin (LMWH), may be considered in the case of recurrent infarction.

CURRENT REVIEW

Bang OY, Seok JM, Kim SG, et al. Ischemic stroke and cancer: stroke severely impacts cancer patients, while cancer increases the number of strokes. *J Clin Neurol* 2011; 7: 53–9.

SUGGESTED READING

Amico L, Caplan LR, Thomas C. Cerebrovascular complications of mucinous cancers. *Neurology* 1989; **39**: 522–6.

Grisold W, Oberndorfer S, Struhal W. Stroke and cancer: a review. *Acta Neurol Scand* 2009; **119**: 1–16.

Kim SG, Hong JM, Kim HY, et al. Ischemic stroke in cancer patients with and without conventional mechanisms: a multicenter study in Korea. *Stroke* 2010; **41**: 798–801.

Rogers LR. Cerebrovascular complications in patients with cancer. *Semin Neurol* 2004; **24**: 453–60.

Schwazbach CJ, Schaefer A, Ebert A, et al. Stroke and cancer: the importance of cancer-associated hypercoagulation as a possible stroke etiology. *Stroke* 2012; **43**(11): 3029–34.

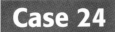

Repeated episodes of weakness and visual loss

Eva Hornberger and Valentin Held

Clinical history

A 60-year-old man was admitted to our stroke unit with dysarthria and left-sided hemiparesis (NIHSS, 3) that started 12 hours earlier. He reported a history of transient episodes with alternating but mostly left-sided weakness and tingling recurring monthly–accompanied by a visual disturbance described as a scotoma– that had been diagnosed as migraine aura without headache. This time, however, worried by the unusually long duration of his symptoms, he came to the emergency room.

Special studies

DWI showed an acute subcortical ischemic lesion in the right centrum semiovale. Additionally, pronounced T2-hyperintense lesions with accentuation were found adjacent to the temporal horns and affecting the extreme capsule (Figure 24.1).

Diagnostic stroke evaluation, including Doppler-/duplex sonography, TTE, and ECG monitoring, was without pathological findings. Neuropsychological evaluation showed mild cognitive deficits (MMSE score, 28). Functional TCD (fTCD) of the posterior cerebral arteries showed no significant alterations of vasomotor reactivity.

Because of the patient's history of migraine aura without headache, the acute ischemic stroke, and the atypical white matter lesions, we suspected CADASIL, which was confirmed by genetic analysis showing a point mutation in the *Notch3* gene. His 40-year-old daughter, who also had migraine with aura has similar T2-hyperintense MRI brain lesions, and was also tested positive for CADASIL.

More Case Studies in Stroke, eds. Michael G. Hennerici, Rolf Kern, Louis R. Caplan, and Kristina Szabo. Published by Cambridge University Press. © Cambridge University Press 2014.

Follow-up

During his hospital stay, the patient had recurring episodes of transient, mainly right-sided sensorimotor hemiparesis and scotoma, in the absence of additional ischemic lesions on follow-up MRI scans. We started the patient on valproate as migraine prophylaxis. Under valproate 1500 mg/d, the attacks gradually decreased and stopped within two weeks. At discharge, there were residual signs including left-sided facial paresis and slight cognitive deficits (NIHSS 2). At the 18-month follow-up examination, the patient reported no additional stroke-like episodes. He was doing well otherwise, with only little progression of his cognitive deficits.

Imaging findings

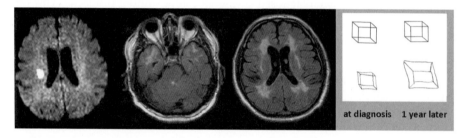

Figure 24.1. DWI shows acute ischemic lesions in the white matter of the left hemisphere. T2-FLAIR detects extensive hyperintense lesions with accentuation adjacent to the temporal horns and affecting the extreme capsule. (An excerpt from the neuropsychological assessment [drawing of a complex object] at the time of diagnosis and one year later.)

Diagnosis

Cerebral autosomal dominant arteriopathy with subcortical infarcts and leuko-encephalopathy (CADASIL).

General remarks

CADASIL is a monogenic cause of ischemic small-vessel disease and stroke in middle-aged individuals. Clinical manifestations include TIAs and strokes (80%), cognitive deficits (50%), migraine with aura (40%), psychiatric disorders (30%), and epilepsy (10%). Migraine characteristics in CADASIL patients show a higher proportion of migraine with aura than in the general population. Visual disturbances are the most prominent aura symptoms whereas transient hemiparesis is rare.

Migrainous infarction, on the other hand, is a rare cause of ischemic stroke in patients who have migraine with aura. It is well defined and characterized by typical aura symptoms as known from previous migraine attacks, with persisting deficits over 60 minutes and showing acute ischemic stroke on imaging. According to epidemiological studies, 0.5%–1.5% of all ischemic strokes are migrainous infarctions.

Special remarks

The clinical history and acute presentation of the patient suggested migrainous infarction. However, the extensive workup revealed CADASIL as the most probable etiology of stroke, therefore excluding formally the diagnosis of migrainous infarction in a strict sense. This finding stresses the necessity of a comprehensive and detailed stroke workup before making the diagnosis of migrainous infarction.

This case reveals the difficulty of interpreting transient neurological symptoms in patients with CADASIL and migraine with aura, as on one hand, ischemic stroke is highly prevalent in CADASIL patients, and on the other hand, CADASIL patients have a higher prevalence of migraine with aura. Acephalic migraine complicates the interpretation even more, as headache, which could help to differentiate between both entities, does not occur. As a further point, this patient presented with atypical aura symptoms, making the diagnosis even more difficult. This case illustrates the complex relationship between migraine, stroke, and CADASIL in an exemplary way: is migraine aura due to brain abnormalities in the context of CADASIL; is stroke a consequence of the vasculopathy due to CADASIL; or is the stroke primarily related to the migraine aura? Temporal lobe white matter lesions are particularly prevalent in CADASIL and may help in the diagnosis.

SUGGESTED READING

Dichgans M, Mayer M, Uttner I, et al. The phenotypic spectrum of CADASIL: clinical findings in 102 cases. *Ann Neurol* 1998; **44**: 731–9.

Laurell K, Artto V, Bendtsen L, et al. Migrainous infarction: a Nordic multicenter study. *Eur J Neurol* 2011; **18**: 1220–6.

Martikainen MH, Roine S. Rapid improvement of a complex migrainous episode with sodium valproate in a patient with CADASIL. *J Headache Pain* 2012; **13**: 95–7.

Vahedi K, Chabriat H, Levy C, et al. Migraine with aura and brain magnetic resonance imaging abnormalities in patients with CADASIL. *Arch Neurol* 2004; **61**: 1237–40.

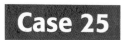

A woman with transient double vision

Philipp Eisele

Clinical history

An 83-year-old woman presented to the emergency room after a transient episode of double vision lasting for about an hour. On the previous day she had suffered an attack of dizziness and had collapsed in the bathroom. She also reported having undergone several dental procedures in the weeks before. Apart from hypertension and hyperlipidemia, medical records revealed hypertrophic cardiomyopathy and calcific aortic valves.

Examination

The neurological examination was normal. She was afebrile; however, cardiac examination showed a systolic murmur.

Neurological scores: NIHSS 0, Barthel 100, mRS 0, GCS 15.

Special studies

An ECG showed normal sinus rhythm; her blood pressure was normal. Emergency MRI was performed, showing multiple acute small embolic lesions scattered in different vascular territories of the brain on DWI, without vessel abnormalities suggestive of a cardiac source of embolism (Figure 25.1A). Laboratory tests showed an elevated CRP of 80 mg/L, while the white blood cell count was normal. Even though infective endocarditis was assumed, emergency TTE remained non-diagnostic; however, TEE on the next day revealed two aortic valve vegetations of 4 mm diameter (Figure 25.1B).

Clinical course

Intravenous antibiotic treatment with a combination of ampicillin and sulbactam was started on day 1 for suspected infective endocarditis. After confirmation by echocardiography and after blood cultures came back positive for

More Case Studies in Stroke, eds. Michael G. Hennerici, Rolf Kern, Louis R. Caplan, and Kristina Szabo.
Published by Cambridge University Press. © Cambridge University Press 2014.

Streptococcus ovis, gentamycin and ceftriaxone were added. After 7 days, the patient was referred to the department of cardiac surgery for an operation. Preoperative assessment included a coronary angiogram to exclude coronary artery disease, and abdominal and chest CT scans to identify a possible primary focus of infection. The patient was referred to a center with extensive experience in cardiac surgery and underwent an operation on day 9 after admission, with replacement of the aortic valve. Antibiotic therapy was continued for 6 weeks; 4 weeks after surgery she was discharged to a rehabilitation facility.

Imaging findings

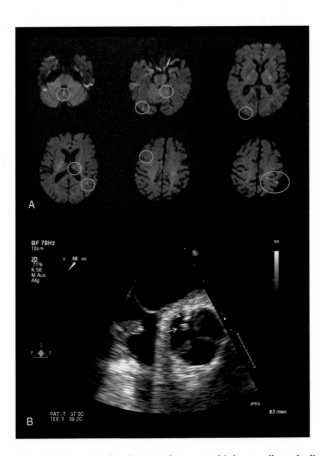

Figure 25.1. (A): diffusion-weighted MRI shows multiple small embolic infarctions in all vascular territories (encircled). (B): transesophageal view of the aortic valve showing vegetations (arrows).

Diagnosis

Disseminated brain embolism in infective endocarditis.

General remarks

Infective endocarditis is an inflammatory process of the inner layer of the heart, usually involving the heart valves, caused by a microbial infection (mostly bacteria – most commonly *Staphylococcus* or *Streptococcus* – but also fungi, or chlamydia). In the past decades, the incidence of infective endocarditis has increased, especially in older patients and is associated with a high mortality of 25%–even higher in specific subgroups. At risk for developing infective endocarditis are injecting drug users, hemodialysis patients, patients with diabetes, and HIV patients. Pre-existing heart disease (especially mitral valve prolapse) and prosthetic heart valves predispose to the development of infective endocarditis. Dental and abdominal procedures and nosocomial infections (via a central venous line) are common routes of infection. Infective endocarditis should be suspected in patients with embolism of unknown origin, fever, sepsis, and a new heart murmur.

Therapy consists of long-term i.v. bactericidal antibiotic therapy, preferably using synergistic drug combinations. About 35%–60% of patients with infective endocarditis will require surgery eventually. Indications for surgery in acute infective endocarditis are based on expert consensus and include development of heart failure, elevated left ventricular end-diastolic or left atrial pressures, and infection with fungi or highly resistant organisms. Surgery also might be considered to prevent recurrent emboli with persistent vegetations under therapy, and very large vegetations. Surgery is performed to remove infectious tissue and repair or replace the affected structures.

Special remarks

Up to 40% of patients with infective endocarditis develop neurological complications, with the most common being septic embolism with ischemic stroke or hemorrhagic infarction. As these may remain asymptomatic, brain MRI should be performed in all patients with infective endocarditis. In a recent study of 85 patients with left-sided infective endocarditis, MRI revealed acute ischemic lesions in 47 (55%), but only 19 developed clinical symptoms. Multiple lesions were present in 77%. Less common complications of infective endocarditis include abscesses, aneurysms, and toxic-metabolic encephalopathies and seizures.

International guidelines advise that patients with stroke due to infective endocarditis should not receive anticoagulants in the acute phase; the use of platelet inhibitors is not recommended. Oral anticoagulants might be replaced by unfractioned heparin for the first two weeks. Infective endocarditis also is a contraindication for thrombolysis. However, diagnosis might not be evident in all cases or established in the narrow time-window for thrombolysis decision. Case studies have reported conflicting outcomes regarding safety and efficacy.

SUGGESTED READING

Habib G, Hoen B, Tornos P, et al. Guidelines on the prevention, diagnosis, and treatment of infective endocarditis (new version 2009): the Task Force on the Prevention, Diagnosis, and Treatment of Infective Endocarditis of the European Society of Cardiology (ESC). *Eur Heart J* 2009; **30**(19): 2369–413.

Okazaki S, Yoshioka D, Sakaguchi M, et al. Acute ischemic brain lesions in infective endocarditis: incidence, related factors, and postoperative outcome. *Cerebrovasc Dis* 2013; **35**(2): 155–62.

Ong E, Mechtouff L, Bernard E, et al. Thrombolysis for stroke caused by infective endocarditis: an illustrative case and review of the literature. *J Neurol* 2013; **260**(5): 1339–42.

Pruitt AA. Neurologic complications of infective endocarditis. *Curr Treat Options Neurol* 2013; **15**(4): 465–76.

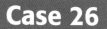
Case 26

Acute myocardial infarction during thrombolysis

Ana Patrícia Antunes, Ruth Geraldes, Tiago Teodoro

Clinical history and examination

An 80-year-old man presented to the emergency department 90 minutes after the sudden onset of slurred speech while gardening. Two days before he had noticed transient slight chest pain. On neurological examination, he was dysarthric, and had a left gaze paresis, a decreased left nasolabial fold, and a drift of his left leg when both lower extremities were held up and straightened (NIHSS 4). An emergency brain CT excluded intracranial hemorrhage and showed no signs of ischemia. The ECG disclosed atrial fibrillation and QS pattern in leads V1–V3, suggestive of an old anteroseptal myocardial infarction. Laboratory evaluation, including hemogram, coagulation, and troponin, was normal.

At that time, our working diagnosis was an acute ischemic stroke and as there were no contraindications, i.v. r-tPA therapy was started 165 minutes after the onset of symptoms (alteplase 0.9 mg/kg body weight: bolus 6.7 mg followed by 60.4 mg in a 60-min infusion). Suddenly, 45 minutes after infusion onset, the patient developed chest pain, anxiety, profuse sweating, facial flushing, and arterial hypertension (180/100 mmHg). Assuming an acute coronary syndrome, intravenous isosorbide dinitrate was initiated immediately. The pain was relieved promptly and blood pressure was controlled. The IVT ended at the expected time and the patient had a slight neurological improvement, regaining lower limb strength but maintaining the left gaze paresis, dysarthria, and mild left facial paresis (NIHSS 3).

In parallel, an urgent ECG disclosed a new 3 mm ST-segment elevation in the inferior leads (DII, DIII, and aVF) and frequent ventricular extrasystoles, and there was an elevation of cardiac biomarkers (troponin I increased from 0.05 ng/mL at baseline to 0.72 ng/mL after thrombolysis [reference value <0.07 ng/mL]). A cardiologist was called and an urgent TTE showed diffuse left ventricular hypokinesis without intracardiac thrombus or valvular vegetations. At this point,

More Case Studies in Stroke, eds. Michael G. Hennerici, Rolf Kern, Louis R. Caplan, and Kristina Szabo.
Published by Cambridge University Press. © Cambridge University Press 2014.

an acute myocardial infarction of the inferior wall with ST-segment elevation was diagnosed. Owing to clinical improvement, the cardiologist deferred percutaneous coronary intervention (PCI) and a single dose of clopidogrel 300 mg and subcutaneous enoxaparin 60 mg were given 90 minutes after r-tPA infusion was stopped.

General history

The patient was an ex-smoker and had hypertension, ischemic heart disease, and chronic obstructive pulmonary disease.

Special studies

Despite neurological improvement, the follow-up brain CT scan (14 hours after thrombolysis) showed a left cerebellar hematoma. The brain MRI, performed two days after thrombolysis, disclosed two acute ischemic lesions in the right MCA and PCA territories and the left cerebellar hematoma (Figure 26.1). Cervical Doppler and TCD examinations and routine laboratory evaluation were normal.

Troponin I values were increased until day 2 after the chest pain (maximum 14.17 ng/mL) and then declined. A second TTE confirmed severe impairment of left ventricular systolic function due to significant ventricular wall hypokinesia but no mural thrombus. A coronary angiogram showed a 60% stenosis in the middle segment of the left anterior descending coronary artery. The coronary arteries supplying the inferior myocardial wall (left circumflex coronary and right coronary arteries) had no atherosclerotic plaques. There was no indication for revascularization treatment.

Imaging findings

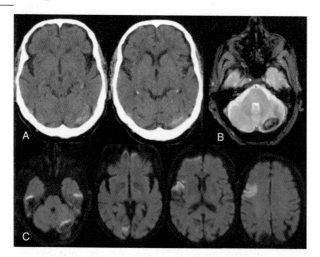

Figure 26.1. (A): Brain CT scan 14 hours after thrombolysis, and (B): T2* brain MRI two days after thrombolysis showing a left cerebellar hematoma. (C): DWI showing two acute ischemic lesions in the right PCA and MCA territories and the left cerebellar hematoma.

Diagnosis

- Cardioembolic ischemic stroke due to non-valvular atrial fibrillation.
- ST-segment elevation acute myocardial infarction during IVT for acute ischemic stroke.
- Asymptomatic intracranial hematoma associated with i.v. thrombolytic therapy and early antiplatelet and anticoagulation treatment.

Follow-up

The patient maintained antiplatelet therapy with aspirin 100 mg from day 2. There was no recurrence of ischemic stroke or chest pain episodes. The follow-up brain CT scan at day 7 after stroke showed partial absorption of the cerebellar hematoma.

There was complete regression of the neurological deficits and he was discharged on the 14th day after admission (NIHSS 0, mRS 0). The start of oral anticoagulation was delayed until day 21 after stroke. One month later he remained asymptomatic.

General remarks

Acute myocardial infarction following administration of i.v. r-tPA for an acute ischemic stroke has been recognized before. There are eight reported cases of patients who developed an acute myocardial infarction in this context, from 10 minutes of r-tPA infusion onset to 15 hours later. This association may have several explanations:

- Systemic thrombolysis for acute ischemic stroke may lead to fragmentation of an underlying cardiac thrombus with subsequent coronary embolization causing myocardial infarction. In fact, in two of the eight patients who developed an acute myocardial infarction after administration of i.v. r-tPA, an unknown intracardiac thrombus was found.
- Acute ischemic stroke may trigger sympathoadrenal activation not only because it is a stressful event but also through lesions in autonomic regulation areas. This can contribute to disruption of cardiovascular physiology–neurogenic heart disease.
- Acute ischemic stroke and acute myocardial infarction may be concurrent manifestations of a systemic atherosclerotic disease.
- A prothrombotic state after thrombolysis for stroke may trigger *in situ* formation of a coronary thrombus in an already unstable atherosclerotic plaque.
- Common etiologies may contribute to concurrent development of stroke and myocardial infarction, such as aortic dissection, large vessel arteritis, endocarditis, or drugs.

In our case, although we could not demonstrate an intracardiac thrombus, the absence of structural coronary artery disease related to the current acute myocardial ischemia suggests either coronary embolism or neurogenic myocardial injury.

Management of myocardial infarction following systemic thrombolysis for an acute ischemic stroke is challenging and has to be individualized. The recommended management of acute myocardial infarction with ST-segment elevation includes reperfusion therapies (PCI or i.v. fibrinolysis) and antiplatelet plus anticoagulation co-therapies (clopidogrel, aspirin, and parenteral anticoagulant therapy). However, in the event of r-tPA administration for acute ischemic stroke, antithrombotic therapies should not be administered for 24 hours, in opposition to the standard treatment of acute myocardial infarction. Urgent primary PCI should be considered in cases of refractory chest pain, persistent ECG changes, or impending cardiovascular failure. Our patient was asymptomatic and hemodynamically stable when he was evaluated by the cardiologist, and therefore primary PCI was postponed. The standard therapy for acute myocardial infarction with clopidogrel plus enoxaparin was considered necessary to salvage the heart, despite an increased risk of hemorrhagic complications. Indeed, this treatment decision was complicated by a cerebellar hematoma that, fortunately, was asymptomatic.

Special remarks

The risk of early recurrent embolism after a cardioembolic stroke has been reported to vary between 0.1% and 1.3% per day during the first two weeks after the initial event. Early re-embolization is associated with a higher in-hospital mortality. After an acute cardioembolic stroke, urgent anticoagulation to prevent early recurrence must be weighed against the risk of brain hemorrhage. The optimal time to start anticoagulation still is controversial. A meta-analysis of randomized controlled trials compared the efficacy and safety of immediate anti-coagulation versus other treatments (aspirin or placebo), focusing exclusively on patients with presumed cardioembolic stroke. Results revealed that early anticoagulation in these patients was associated with a significant increase in symptomatic intracranial bleeding, a nonsignificant reduction in recurrent stroke within seven to 14 days, and a similar rate of death or disability at the end of follow-up (at least three months). Therefore, aspirin therapy is recommended formally for all patients with acute ischemic stroke, based on high-quality evidence in favor of antiplatelet therapy and lack of evidence to support routine use of early anticoagulation. However, it has to be stressed that only one trial (Cerebral Embolism Study Group–CESG) out of the seven individual studies included in the meta-analysis was designed specifically for cardioembolic strokes, and all other trials excluded patients with a clear indication for anticoagulation. Therefore, some experts recommend immediate anticoagulation in selected cardioembolic strokes, such as those associated with high-risk cardiac conditions, who are underrepresented in the clinical trials. Acute anticoagulation in this setting has to be individualized and should be considered when the risk of hemorrhagic complications is low (small infarcts, controlled arterial hypertension, and no evidence of hemorrhage on imaging).

In our case, there was a high cardioembolic risk due to atrial fibrillation and recent myocardial infarction, but the presence of an acute brain hematoma further complicated the decision on anticoagulation timing. Limited data are available to guide the management of anticoagulation in patients with ischemic stroke and hemorrhagic infarction. There has been near unanimity about avoiding or discontinuing anticoagulation if hemorrhagic infarction is present, due to the fear of transforming the hemorrhagic infarction into hematoma with clinical deterioration and death. However, few studies have reported a favorable clinical course in selected patients with hemorrhagic infarction kept on anticoagulation after hemorrhagic infarction was visualized on CT.

Concerning anticoagulant therapy for secondary prevention in this patient with atrial fibrillation, a CHA2DS2–VASc score of 6 indicates a high risk of stroke (estimated risk of 9.8% per year) requiring oral anticoagulation, and a HAS–BLED score of 3 indicates increased risk of major bleeding on anticoagulation, sufficient to justify caution or more regular review. Taking all this into account, we decided to postpone anticoagulation initiation for three weeks.

SUGGESTED READING

Arboix A, García-Eroles L, Oliveres M, Massons JB, Targa C. Clinical predictors of early embolic recurrence in presumed cardioembolic stroke. *Cerebrovasc Dis* 1998; **8**: 345–53.

Caplan LR, Manning WJ. *Brain Embolism*. New York, NY: Informa Healthcare, 2006.

Mehdiratta M, Murphy C, Al-Harthi A, Teal PA. Myocardial infarction following tPA for acute stroke. *Can J Neurol Sci* 2007; **34**: 417–20.

Meissner W, Lempert T, Saeuberlich-Knigge S, Bocksch W, Pape UF. Fatal embolic myocardial infarction after systemic thrombolysis for stroke. *Cerebrovasc Dis* 2006; **22**: 213–14.

Paciaroni M, Agnelli G, Micheli S, Caso V. A meta-analysis of randomized controlled trials efficacy and safety of anticoagulant treatment in acute cardioembolic stroke. *Stroke* 2007; **38**: 423–30.

Pessin MS, Estol CJ, Lafranchise F, Caplan LR. Safety of anticoagulation after hemorrhagic infarction. *Neurology* 1993; **43**: 1298–303.

Santos N, Serrão M, Silva B, et al. Acute myocardial infarction after thrombolytic treatment of acute ischemic stroke. *Rev Port Cardiol* 2009; **28**: 1161–6.

Saxena R, Lewis S, Berge E, Sandercock PA, Koudstaal PJ. Risk of early death and recurrent stroke and effect of heparin in 3169 patients with acute ischemic stroke and atrial fibrillation in the International Stroke Trial. *Stroke* 2001; **32**: 2333–7.

Sweta A, Sejal S, Prakash S, Vinay C, Shirish H. Acute myocardial infarction following intravenous tissue plasminogen activator for acute ischemic stroke: an unknown danger. *Ann Indian Acad Neurol* 2010; **13**: 64–6.

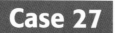

A misleading ca(u)se of cerebral microbleeds

Sofie De Blauwe, Katlijn Schotsmans, and Gregory Helsen

Clinical history

A 56-year-old woman with a history of hypertension was admitted to the emergency department because of paresis and paresthesia of the right leg, accompanied by a light headache. She presented approximately 24 hours after symptom onset. For the hypertension, she was being treated with a beta-blocker (nebivolol 2.5 mg/day), an angiotensin-converting enzyme (ACE)-inhibitor blocker (irbesartan 300 mg/day), and a diuretic (hydrochlorothiazide 12.5 mg), with moderate results. Her father had Parkinson's disease. Her mother survived breast cancer.

Non-contrast-enhanced CT showed an intracerebral hemorrhage (ICH) in the left frontal lobe with some surrounding edema (Figure 27.1A). On MRI, T2* images showed, in addition, multiple "microbleeds" (Figure 27.1B,D,F). Differential diagnosis at that time was either hypertensive vasculopathy or cerebral amyloid angiopathy (CAA). Within a few days, the patient recovered completely. Her hypertension was treated and she was discharged. Follow-up consultation and MRI were scheduled three months later.

Two months later, the patient was readmitted to our hospital. She now presented with a right hemiparesis and mild expressive aphasia. Noncontrast-enhanced CT now showed multiple spontaneous hyperdense lesions in the left temporoparietal region (Figure 27.1C). There was partial resorption of the hemorrhage in the left frontal lobe. We conducted further examinations.

Examination

Clinical examination on this admission showed dysarthria, slight expressive aphasia, right facial palsy, and paresis of the right leg. The patient was obese and hypertensive (with an arterial blood pressure of 156/96 mmHg upon admission).

Special studies

Routine laboratory results were normal, except for elevated alkaline phosphatase (101 U/L) and gamma-glutamyl transferase (190 U/L). On transesophageal

More Case Studies in Stroke, eds. Michael G. Hennerici, Rolf Kern, Louis R. Caplan, and Kristina Szabo.
Published by Cambridge University Press. © Cambridge University Press 2014.

echocardiography (TEE), there was no evidence of endocarditis. Cerebral angiography showed no causative lesions. The patient underwent a study protocol 11C-PiB-PET brain scan as she fulfilled the Boston criteria for probable CAA. The result was normal and no increased amount of amyloid deposits was detected.

A new MRI was performed and showed that during these two months, new lesions had developed (Figure 27.1E), and that several lesions present on the first MRI had grown substantially and acted as space-occupying lesions, some with surrounding edema (Figure 27.1G). Additionally, some lesions were spontaneously hyperintense on T1. There was contrast enhancement on T1 with gadolinium. A whole body FDG-PET scan revealed a hyperintense locus in the brain in the left parietotemporal region, on the gallbladder, and on the seventh thoracic vertebra, suggestive of metastases. Taking the characteristics of the lesions into account, we suspected melanoma. Upon thorough clinical examination, there was one mole on the left thigh that looked suspicious. A combined biopsy of a brain metastasis and the skin lesion were performed. These confirmed the diagnosis of melanoma.

Imaging findings

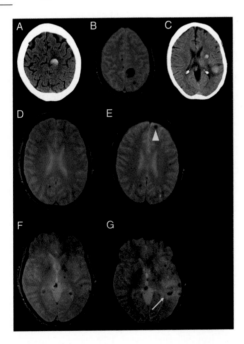

Figure 27.1. Top row: hyperdense lesion in a noncontrast-enhanced CT performed at the first presentation with paresis of the right leg (A); T2* MRI showing the same lesion, with several other microbleeds (B); and non-contrast-enhanced CT performed two months later (C). Middle and bottom row: base T2* MRI (D,F) compared with the T2* MRI upon the second episode (right), showing a new lesion (arrowhead) (E) and substantial growth with surrounding edema of an existing lesion (arrow) (G).

Diagnosis

The patient was diagnosed with malignant melanoma with metastases of the brain, vertebrae, and gallbladder.

Follow-up

We referred the patient to the oncology department for treatment. She received both cranial radiotherapy and several courses of chemotherapy (in total, six administrations of dacarbazine every two weeks, and because of tumor progression under this regime, three courses of ipilimumab). In between, she had an episode of acute paraplegia due to medullary compression of the metastasis that involved the seventh thoracic vertebra. Tumorectomy was successful. Eventually she developed melena from a metastasis to the small intestine and passed away 18 months after the initial diagnosis.

General remarks

Microbleeds are seen in 11.1%–23.5% of the population. The most common causes are hypertensive vasculopathy and CAA, both associated with a different distribution pattern of the lesions. In hypertension, lesions are predominantly seen in the thalamus, basal ganglia, brainstem, and cerebellum, whereas in CAA, there is a lobar distribution, with most lesions found in the posterior cortical regions [1]. In CAA, beta-amyloid deposits in the media and adventitia of small arteries and capillaries of the leptomeninges and the cerebral cortex. The Pittsburgh compound-B (PIB) is a thioflavin derivative that ligands to this beta-amyloid. PIB binding is increased moderately in most patients with probable CAA-related ICH [2]. Microbleeds need to be differentiated from several mimics: calcification, iron deposition, cavernous malformations, and melanoma metastasis.

Special remarks

Of all brain metastases, 75% are caused by lung cancer, breast cancer, or melanoma. Brain metastases of melanoma have distinctive features on MRI. They frequently are spontaneously T1 hyperintense and T2* hypointense. They usually show contrast enhancement and some edema. It is thought that they display these features because of the paramagnetic properties of the melanin pigment and their frequent bleeding complications [3]. The spontaneous hyperdensity on CT is thought to be caused by bleeding as well.

REFERENCES

1. Greenberg SM, Vernooij MW, Cordonnier C, et al. Cerebral microbleeds: a guide to detection and interpretation. *Lancet Neurol* 2009; **8**: 165–74.
2. Ly JV, Donnan GA, Villemagne VL, et al. 11C-PIB binding is increased in patients with cerebral amyloid angiopathy-related hemorrhage. *Neurology* 2010; **74**: 487–93.
3. Gaviani P, Mullins ME, Braga TA, et al. Improved detection of metastatic melanoma by T2*-weighted imaging. *Am J Neuroradiol* 2006; **27**: 605–8.

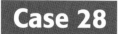

A psychiatrist battered by the sea

Louis R. Caplan

Clinical history

A 51-year-old eccentric psychiatrist became bored and restless during a psychiatric meeting away from home. He left the meeting and rented a sailboat despite
warnings that a storm was approaching. The winds became very strong and he felt
"battered by the sea." The sailboat he rented was swept out of control and he had
to grip strongly to hold on to prevent falling. Later that same day, he developed
pain in his neck and he had a headache. He had a momentary brief vision of a
scintillating waterfall to his left. A week later, during which he continued to have
an occipital headache, he again had a similar visual illusion to his left. Two days
later, he suddenly developed ptosis and left limb clumsiness. Nine years previously, during extreme stress, he had a left hemiparesis due to a right hypertensive
putaminal hemorrhage, but his blood pressure was well controlled after that.

Examination

On examination, his blood pressure was 125/80 mmHg. Results of cognitive tests,
including drawing, copying, and ability to revisualize were normal. Visual fields
were normal. The right eyelid was severely ptotic. The eyes diverged, with the right
resting down and out. He had a left gaze palsy accompanied by tortional nystagmus in a clockwise rotation that was more obvious in the left eye. He had little up-
gaze. On attempted down-gaze, the left eye dipped below the right and showed
prominent tortional nystagmus. Pupils were 4.5 mm and reacted normally. The
left limbs were clumsy but not weak. Left limb reflexes were increased, and the left
plantar response was extensor. Gait was wide-based.

Special studies

DWI showed a right paramedian midbrain infarct, and a small right paramedian
thalamic infarct was shown on FLAIR. He had a small slit cavity in the right

More Case Studies in Stroke, eds. Michael G. Hennerici, Rolf Kern, Louis R. Caplan, and Kristina Szabo.
Published by Cambridge University Press. © Cambridge University Press 2014.

putamen that represented his old putaminal hemorrhage. MRA showed a dilated proximal segment of the right PCA, followed by a string-like lumen. Later MRA scans showed normalization of the right PCA lesion (Figure 28.1).

Follow-up

The neurological deficit improved significantly within two hours after therapy.

Imaging findings

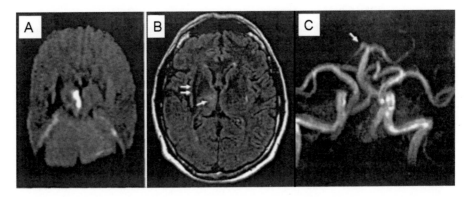

Figure 28.1. (A): DWI demonstrated an acute ischemic paramedian midbrain lesion on the right. (B): T2 FLAIR showed an additional small paramedian thalamic infarct on the right (white arrow); there was a small slit cavity in the right putamen (two white arrows) representing the chronic putaminal hemorrhage. (C): a dilated proximal segment of the right PCA, followed by a string-like lumen (white arrow), was shown on MRA.

Diagnosis

Dissection of the PCA.

Remarks

The patient had developed a dissection of his right PCA. This occurred during a storm with sudden neck and head movements. The manifestations were headache, transient left visual field TIAs followed by an infarct in the distribution of the right PCA in its proximal portion. The penetrating arteries to the midbrain and thalamus were affected, causing a midbrain infarct. The major clinical signs were oculomotor–a left conjugate gaze palsy, vertical ophthalmoplegia, and torsional nystagmus. In addition, there was slight left limb ataxia.

Intracranial arterial dissections are much less common than those that affect the cervical carotid and VAs. In my experience, they are often provoked by sudden movements as are neck dissections. Intracranial dissections most often involve the carotid arteries in their intracranial portions, and the intracranial VAs. PCA dissections are quite rare.

SUGGESTED READING

Caplan LR. Dissections of brain-supplying arteries. *Nat Clin Pract Neurol* 2008; **4**(1): 34–42.

Caplan LR, Estol CJ, Massaro AR. Dissection of the posterior cerebral arteries. *Arch Neurol* 2005; **62**: 1138–43.

Chaves C, Estol C, Esnaola MM, et al. Spontaneous intracranial internal carotid artery dissection. *Arch Neurol* 2002; **59**: 977–81.

Estol CJ, Caplan LR. Intracranial arterial dissections. In Caplan LR, van Gijn (eds.), *Stroke Syndromes*, 3rd edn. Cambridge: Cambridge University Press, 2012; 566–73.

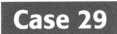

Severe migraine with double vision

Louis R. Caplan

Case history

A 54-year-old man was seen because of an unusual occurrence of an ICH. He was a truck driver and had had a 25-year history of complex migraine attacks. During some attacks, he would become confused. In one, he saw a black dot on the right and then lost some vision within the right visual field; when he tried to read, he had difficulty reading to the right. In one episode, he lost vision, his right hand became shaky, and he had some difficulty speaking. In other episodes, he had problems reading and writing and some difficulty understanding spoken language. In a few of the attacks, his right arm and hand felt strange. He also had had frequent headaches, some of which were behind the right eye. Headaches often preceded or followed the prolonged attacks, which typically lasted from 15 minutes to an hour or longer.

On the day of the stroke, after attending a movie he ate ice cream and developed a dull throbbing headache. The headache was in the left occipital area and gradually became severe. Shortly after the headache eased, he began to have difficulty with vision; he described double vision with the objects seen one beside and above the other in an oblique relationship, most apparent in the right visual field. He remembers transiently having difficulty speaking shortly thereafter. He was evaluated at a nearby hospital, where he was found to have normal blood pressure, and a CT scan showed a left temporo-occipital ICH (Figure 29.1).

Since then, he often would see an object that would drift off to the right; if he saw someone and he or she moved, he would still continue to see the individual. At times, if he heard something, he would continue to hear it afterward. These experiences were brief, lasting less than a minute. He denied any other major medical problems or drug abuse. He has never had high blood pressure and was not aware of any excess bleeding or clotting disorder.

More Case Studies in Stroke, eds. Michael G. Hennerici, Rolf Kern, Louis R. Caplan, and Kristina Szabo. Published by Cambridge University Press. © Cambridge University Press 2014.

Examination

On neurological examination, his visual fields were normal to confrontation; he was slow in reading and made spelling and grammatical errors in writing. He had no motor, sensory, or reflex abnormalities. His pulse was 72 beats/min, blood pressure 125/80 mmHg.

Special studies

An MRI was performed several years after the initial hemorrhage. The T2* gradient-recalled echo, susceptibility-weighted sequence showed a smaller region of hemosiderin (Figure 29.1). Digital angiography was performed and was entirely normal.

Imaging findings

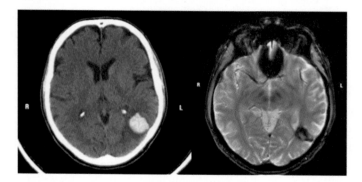

Figure 29.1. CT of the brain showed an acute left temporo-occipital ICH (left). T2* susceptibility-weighted images (right) detected a smaller region of hemosiderin representing the chronic hemorrhagic lesion.

Diagnosis

Migraine-related brain hemorrhage.

Remarks

The most likely diagnosis is a migraine-related brain hemorrhage. Hemorrhage into brain parenchyma has been reported occasionally after migraine attacks. The first report was by Dunning who described the case of a young normotensive woman who developed a right ICH on the fourth day of a severe migraine attack. Cole and Aube reported three women who developed ICH after severe migraine headaches. In one of their patients who had left paresthesias, a slight left hemiparesis, and a severe headache, a CT scan during the severe headache with complicated migraine was normal. She then developed a severe left hemiplegia and stupor and a repeat CT scan showed a large right frontal lobar hemorrhage that was decompressed surgically. The other two patients also developed lobar hemorrhages after their severe migraine headache had subsided. Angiography in all of the patients revealed regions of arterial vasoconstriction. In one patient, the narrowing of the extracranial ICA probably was due to a dissection. The authors and I posit that vascular injury to arterioles and capillaries had occurred during the migraine attacks, which were all characterized by angiographically documented vasoconstriction. When the attacks and vasoconstriction subsided, reperfusion of the previously ischemic capillary and arteriolar bed led to hemorrhage. Reperfusion hemorrhage has been shown in other circumstances such as after embolic brain infarction.

SUGGESTED READING

Caplan LR. Intracerebral hemorrhage, revisited. *Neurology* 1988; **38**: 624–6.

Cole AJ, Aube M. Migraine with vasospasm and delayed intracerebral hemorrhage. *Arch Neurol* 1990; **47**: 53–6.

Dunning HS. Intracranial and extracranial vascular accidents in migraine. *Arch Neurol Psychiatr* 1942; **48**: 396–406.

Gautier JC, Majdalani A, Juillard JB, Carmi AR. Cerebral hemorrhage in migraine. *Rev Neurol* 1993; **149**(6–7): 407–10.

Gokhale S, Ghoshal S, Lahotti SA, Caplan LR. An uncommon cause of intracerebral hemorrhage in a healthy truck driver. *Arch Neurol* 2012; **69**(11): 1500–3.

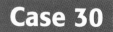

Case 30

Another young woman with infertility

Markus Stürmlinger

Clinical history

A 35-year-old woman was transferred to our emergency room from a community hospital where she had developed fluctuating abnormalities of speech and right hand and face weakness.

Family members reported that she was taking fertility medication. She had been advised by the fertility clinic to drink sufficient amounts of water. She had complained about a severe headache since the day before and had initially gone to the hospital for fear of dehydration as she was not able to drink adequately.

Examination

On admission, the patient was awake and alert. She was mute except for the word "yes"; she had fairly good speech comprehension. She had a severe brachiofacial hemiparesis on the right side.

Neurological scores: NIHSS 14, mRS 5.

Medical history

The patient was undergoing infertility treatment and had received one cycle of ovulation induction with the administration of 10 000 IU of human chorionic gonadotropin ten days earlier. Before that she had received a single-dose of a gonadotropin-releasing hormone analog, followed by daily doses of follicle stimulating hormone and luteinizing hormone for 12 days. Two days before her stroke, she was diagnosed with mild ovarian hyperstimulation syndrome (OHSS) and was given a prophylaxis with low molecular weight heparin (clexane 40 mg/day).

More Case Studies in Stroke, eds. Michael G. Hennerici, Rolf Kern, Louis R. Caplan, and Kristina Szabo. Published by Cambridge University Press. © Cambridge University Press 2014.

She was a non-smoker and had no previous hypertension. There was no family history of arterial or venous thromboembolic disease. She had a history of migraine, but she reported that she had been pain-free for four months. She was taking 50 µg levothyroxine/day for hypothyroidism.

Special studies

The laboratory findings when seen in the emergency room showed an elevated white blood cell count ($21\,300 \times 10^9$/L), reduced sodium (129 mmol/L) and elevated potassium (4.9 mmol/L) levels. Platelet count (398×10^9/L) and hemoglobin (164 g/L) were slightly elevated. Ultrasound examination showed enlarged ovaries and also revealed a small pleural effusion.

Emergency MRI showed a left subcortical hyperacute stroke with a DWI/PWI mismatch and occlusion of the proximal left MCA (Figure 30.1). IVT was started while the patient was transferred to the angiography suite for intra-arterial thrombectomy.

Follow-up

Within three days following complete interventional MCA recanalization, the patient improved to an NIHSS of 1. No sources of a potential cardiac cause of embolism were identified (ECG monitoring/echocardiography). Further diagnostic testing for coagulopathies showed a significant level of antiphospholipid antibodies and anti-β2–glycoprotein 1 antibodies indicating antiphospholipid syndrome.

Imaging findings

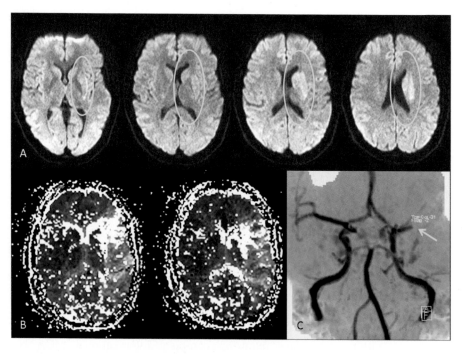

Figure 30.1. (A): DWI at presentation shows faint hyperintense signal in the left basal ganglia indicating hyperacute stroke. (B): Area of hypoperfusion on PWI exceeds the DWI lesion, with involvement of nearly the complete left MCA territory with frontal accentuation including Broca's area. (C): MRA shows occlusion of the proximal left MCA.

Diagnosis

Ovarian hyperstimulation syndrome plus antiphospholipid antibody syndrome and stroke.

General remarks

OHSS is an iatrogenic complication of controlled ovarian stimulation, and is associated with a range of clinical symptoms from mild to moderate features with nausea or ascites, and severe to critical cases with an increased risk of thromboembolic events, acute renal failure, liver dysfunction, ovarian rupture, or manifestations of an adult respiratory distress syndrome. Severe OHSS occurs in approximately 1.4% of all hyperstimulation cycles. Inducing a large number of follicles prior to in vitro fertilization leads to enlargement of ovaries causing abdominal distension. In response to elevated levels of human chorionic gonadotropin, the capillary permeability increases – mediated by vascular endothelial growth factor, inflammatory mediators, and the renin–angiotensin–aldosterone system. Subsequent vascular effusion of protein-rich fluid may lead to ascites and pleural effusions. Young age, allergies, and the polycystic ovary syndrome are risk factors for developing an OHSS. Hyperviscosity, hemoconcentration, and reduced venous return predispose to thromboembolic events, which are reported in the venous system primarily.

Special remarks

Cerebral infarction in OHSS is rare, but most cases reported had an occlusion of large arterial branches resulting in severe ischemic stroke. In the majority of these patients, comorbidities predisposing to thromboembolic events were identified: hypercoagulable states, such as antiphospholipid antibody syndrome, antithrombin III deficiency, or activated protein C resistance; continuous human chorionic gonadotropin levels or sensivity, due to polycystic ovaries or an ongoing pregnancy; or vascular spasms as in one patient with a history of migraine. Therefore, women undergoing infertility treatment who have a personal or family history of thrombosis or thromboembolism should undergo screening for coagulopathies.

SUGGESTED READING

Cluroe AD, Synek BJ. A fatal case of ovarian hyperstimulation syndrome with cerebral infarction. *Pathology* 1995; **27**(4): 344–6.

Davies AJ, Patel B. Hyperstimulation–brain attack. *Br J Radiol* 1999; **72**: 923–4.

Elford K, Leader A, Wee R, Stys PK. Stroke in ovarian hyperstimulation syndrome in early pregnancy treated with intra-arterial rt-PA. *Neurology* 2002; **59**: 1270–2.

Fiedler K, Ezcurra D. Predicting and preventing ovarian hyperstimulation syndrome (OHSS): the need for individualized not standardized treatment. *Reprod Biol Endocrinol* 2012; **10**: 32.

Song TJ, Lee SY, Oh SH, Lee KY. Multiple cerebral infarctions associated with polycystic ovaries and ovarian hyperstimulation syndrome. *Eur Neurol* 2008; **59**: 76–8.

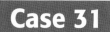

Man with bilateral hypoglossal palsy

Bettina Anders

Clinical history

A 74-year-old, previously healthy man presented with sudden paresthesia of his right lower jaw, difficulties chewing and swallowing, slurred speech, as well as a severe right-sided headache. He also reported excessive coughing during the previous two weeks, diagnosed as bronchitis.

Examination

Neurological examination upon arrival showed a Horner's syndrome on the right and right hypoglossal nerve palsy with deviation of the tongue to the right and dysarthria. Laboratory examination showed an elevated CRP of 148 mg/dl.

Neurological scores: NIHSS 2, mRS 2, GCS 15.

Follow-up/special studies

Initial MRI of the brain and cerebral vessels as well as CSF analysis were normal. On day 4, the patient's symptoms progressed: he developed bilateral hypoglossal nerve palsy with grossly impaired tongue mobility, severe dysarthria, hypophonia, dysphagia, and hypersalivation due to impaired swallowing. Repeat MRI was ordered. There were no acute ischemic lesions, but a thickened wall of both distal ICAs resulting from intramural hematoma without hemodynamic obstruction of the vessel lumen was detected (Figure 31.1). Enteral feeding through a percutaneous endoscopic gastrostomy tube was necessary. The patient was transferred to rehabilitation. On follow-up examinations in our outpatient department the patient had a gradual and slow recovery of symptoms. After a year, there was only slight residual dysarthria and hypophonia; however, he still complained about hypersalivation.

More Case Studies in Stroke, eds. Michael G. Hennerici, Rolf Kern, Louis R. Caplan, and Kristina Szabo. Published by Cambridge University Press. © Cambridge University Press 2014.

Imaging findings

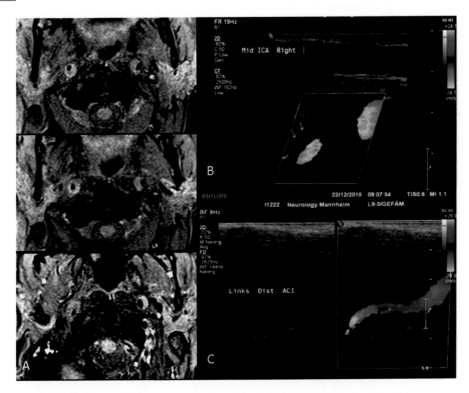

Figure 31.1. (A): Transverse MRI shows an intramural hematoma (arrows) in both distal ICAs as hyperintense signal on fat-saturated T1-weighted images. (B): Transverse ultrasound section of the right ICA, and (C): longitudinal ultrasound section of the left ICA, demonstrate hypoechoic thickening in both vessels (normal vessel lumen, yellow dotted line).

Diagnosis

Bilateral hypoglossal nerve palsy and right Horner's syndrome caused by bilateral carotid artery dissection.

General remarks

Clinical features of arterial dissection, with or without additional focal cerebral ischemic symptoms, include (head–face–neck) pain, Horner's syndrome, tinnitus, and cranial nerve palsy. Patients with these focal signs have been reported to have an eccentric position of the hematoma more commonly. If the extracranial portion of the ICA is affected, cranial nerve palsy is reported to occur in 12% of cases. The hypoglossal nerve is involved most frequently (in 5%) with or without involvement of the cranial nerves XI, X, and IX. A local mechanism of nerve injury by the expanding vessel wall due to the hematoma or by compression of feeder vessels is believed to result in nerve palsy. Interestingly, hypoglossal nerve palsy–without brainstem ischemia–has been reported to occur in VA dissection as well, as vertebral branches supply mainly the proximal cisternal portion of the hypoglossal nerve.

Special remarks

Bilateral simultaneous hypoglossal palsy as a result of bilateral acute ICA dissection without stroke is very rare. In the present case, shear forces due to heavy coughing may have been the triggering factor for the dissections.

SUGGESTED READING

Caplan LR, Gonzalez RG, Buonanno FS. Case 18–2012: a 35-year-old man with neck pain, hoarseness, and dysphagia. *N Engl J Med* 2012; **366**: 2306–13.

Guidetti D, Pisanello A, Giovanardi F, et al. Spontaneous carotid dissection presenting lower cranial nerve palsies. *J Neurol Sci* 2001; **184**(2): 203–7.

Lanczik O, Szabo K, Hennerici M, Gass A. Multiparametric MRI and ultrasound findings in patients with internal carotid artery dissection. *Neurology* 2005; **65**(3): 469–71.

Mahadevappa K, Chacko T, Nair AK. Isolated unilateral hypoglossal nerve palsy due to vertebral artery dissection. *Clin Med Res* 2012; **10**(3): 127–30.

Mokri B, Silbert PL, Schievink WI, et al. Cranial nerve palsy in spontaneous dissection of the extracranial internal carotid artery. *Neurology* 1996; **46**: 356–9.

Olzowy B, Lorenzl S, Guerkov R. Bilateral and unilateral internal carotid artery dissection causing isolated hypoglossal nerve palsy: a case report and review of the literature. *Eur Arch Otorhinolaryngol* 2006; **263**(4): 390–3.

Sturzenegger M, Huber P. Cranial nerve palsies in spontaneous carotid artery dissection. *J Neurol Neurosurg Psychiatry* 1993; **56**(11): 1191–9.

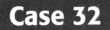

Thoracic pain and right hemispheric syndrome

Nadja Meyer

Clinical history

A 55-year-old man reported an episode of acute severe retrosternal chest pain during work. In the ambulance, he received heparin and aspirin i.v. for suspected acute coronary syndrome. On the way to the hospital, he was pain free but developed an acute left hemiparesis. In the emergency room, systemic thrombolysis with r-tPA was started after exclusion of ICH on CT. Initial 12-lead ECG showed a normal sinus rhythm without ischemic features. Laboratory studies showed an elevated d-dimer value of >32 mg/L (normal range, 0–0.5 mg/L), while high-sensitive troponin 1 was normal (<0.015 µg/L). His neurological symptoms started to improve after approximately 30 minutes, but at this time, he once again reported severe thoracic pain.

The patient's medical history was non-contributory, except for smoking.

Examination

Neurological examination upon arrival to the emergency room and 50 minutes after the onset of symptoms showed a right gaze deviation and gaze preference, complete left homonymous hemianopia, dysarthria, sensorimotor syndrome with brachiofacial accentuation, including hemiplegia of the left arm, and a severe hemiparesis of the left leg. His heart rate was 54 bpm and systolic blood pressure 160 mmHg.

Neurological scores: NIHSS 13, Barthel 5, GCS 15.

Special studies

Pre-thrombolysis cranial CT showed a hyperdense right MCA. Extra- and intracranial ultrasound confirmed a dampened flow signal in the right MCA and showed findings suggestive of extensive dissection of the right common carotid artery (Figure 32.1), the right external carotid artery and ICA, and the right VA.

More Case Studies in Stroke, eds. Michael G. Hennerici, Rolf Kern, Louis R. Caplan, and Kristina Szabo. Published by Cambridge University Press. © Cambridge University Press 2014.

Follow-up

After the ultrasound examination, thrombolysis was discontinued because of strongly suspected dissection of the aorta. At this time, tearing chest pain had returned, he became pale and sweaty and was transferred to the ICU. There was unequal blood pressure between the right and left arm and he became hypotensive. On TTE, a dissection membrane in the posterior part of the ascending aorta was visible; a pericardial effusion was not found. Chest CT confirmed thoracic dissection of the aorta classified as Stanford type A (Figure 32.2), extending from the ascending aorta to the aortic bifurcation, involving the brachiocephalic trunk, the right carotid artery and the VAs, and the superior mesenteric and left renal arteries. During preparation for emergency vascular surgery, the patient became asystole. Resuscitation attempts were unsuccessful and the patient died a few hours after the initial onset of symptoms.

Imaging findings

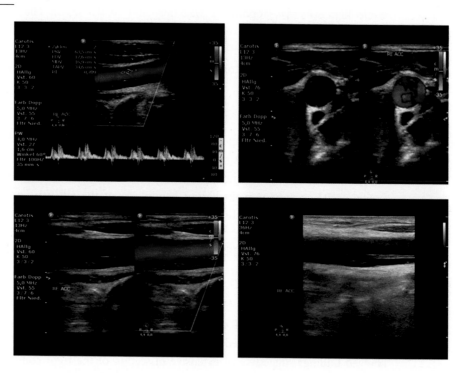

Figure 32.1. Top row: duplex ultrasound of the right common carotid artery in the longitudinal plane on the left shows anterograde flow with typical systolic deceleration, and in the axial plane, anterograde flow in red, and flap in blue (right). Bottom row: intimal flap separating the true and false vessel lumina.

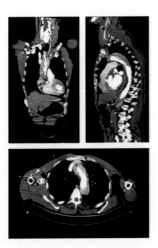

Figure 32.2. Postcontrast chest CT show the dilated aorta with an unopacified false lumen.

Diagnosis

Fatal aortic dissection presenting with acute ischemic stroke.

General remarks

Aortic dissection is a rare and potentially life-threatening disease. It is caused by a disruption of the aortic intima and media with propagation of a "false lumen" within the media. Normally, it presents with sudden and severe pain in the chest and back, and progression of the dissection process by spreading of the pain to abdomen and legs. Sometimes, there is a pain-free interval, lasting from hours to days, and the following return of pain usually signals imminent rupture. About 20% of patients do not report any significant pain. Cerebral ischemia occurs in about 5%–30% of aortic dissections and is caused by occlusion of the common carotid artery by mural hematoma or artery-to-artery embolism from a thrombus developed on the intimal surface of the dissected artery.

The most common risk factor for aortic dissection is chronic systemic hypertension, followed by connective tissue diseases such as Marfans syndrome and Ehlers–Danlos syndrome, cystic media necrosis and bicuspid aortic valve. Aortic dissections can be classified using one of two systems, the Stanford and the DeBakey systems, which both describe anatomical criteria and discriminate the involvement of the ascending aorta. The Stanford system is divided into type A, involving the ascending aorta, and type B, affecting the aorta distal to the subclavian artery. The DeBakey system is more precise: type I originates in the ascending aorta and propagates to the descending vessel, type II is limited to the ascending aorta, and type III to the descending part. Proximal dissections are treated usually with emergent surgical repair; distal ones can be managed conservatively with medical control of blood pressure and radiological monitoring.

Special remarks

In the era of thrombolysis, aortic dissection manifesting as cerebral infarction confronts the clinician with a special diagnostic problem. Especially in cases as this one with the neurological symptoms occurring in the pain-free period, the diagnosis of aortic dissection may be masked and considerably delayed. Important clinical clues that should alert stroke physicians are:

- Chest pain, shock-like symptoms, severe hypotension in patients with hypertension.
- Differences in blood pressure between both arms, asymmetrical pulses, cardiac murmur.
- Widened mediastinum on plain X-ray.

In case studies of patients with stroke or myocardial infarction treated with thrombolysis, who had unrecognized aortic dissection, therapy may have contributed to poor outcome by causing or worsening complications such as ICH, extension of the dissection into the pericardium with subsequent cardiac tamponade, intrapleural hemorrhage, and aortic rupture.

SUGGESTED READING

Cook J, Aeschlimann S, Fuh A, et al. Aortic dissection presenting as concomitant stroke and STEMI. *J Human Hypertens* 2007; **21**: 818–21.

Estrera A, Garami Z, Miller CC, et al. Acute type A aortic dissection complicated by stroke: can immediate repair be performed safely? *J Thorac Cardiovasc Surg* 2006; **132**: 1404–8.

Fessler AJ, Alberts MJ. Stroke treatment with tissue plasminogen activator in the setting of aortic dissection. *Neurology* 2000; **54**: 1010.

Gaul C, Dietrich W, Erbguth FJ. Neurological symptoms in aortic dissection: a challenge for neurologists. *Cerebrovasc Dis* 2008; **26**: 1–8.

Grupper M, Eran A, Shifrin A. Ischemic stroke, aortic dissection, and thrombolytic therapy–the importance of basic clinical skills. *J Gen Intern Med* 2007; **22**: 1370–3.

Iguchi Y, Kazumi K, Sakai K, et al. Hyper-acute stroke patients associated with aortic dissection. *Intern Med* 2010; **49**: 543–7.

Severe gait disorder in a 38-year-old man

Tilman Menzel and Rolf Kern

Clinical history

A 38-year-old man was referred to our department with a gait disorder that had been slowly progressive over approximately two months. Although detailed history of the onset and progression of symptoms was difficult, the onset seemed to be gradual. The patient did not consult a physician until he was hardly able to walk independently and he fell twice at home.

Examination

On initial examination, he had slight brachiofacial hemiparesis as well as spastic paraparesis, especially of the right and proximal lower extremity. The tendon reflexes of the right leg were increased. Babinski's sign was positive and ankle clonus was present bilaterally. Foremost, the patient's gait was severely spastic-ataxic, and he had to use a walking frame for even short distances.

Special studies

Brain MRI showed disseminated bilateral subcortical DWI- and T2-hyperintense lesions, compatible with multiple acute ischemic lesions (Figure 33.1). MRA showed severe narrowing of the left MCA and moderate stenosis of the right MCA. Findings were confirmed by TCD ultrasound. On spinal MRI, the spinal meninges enhanced after contrast agent without any obvious parenchymatous cord lesion. CSF analysis revealed a pleocytosis with 467 lympho-, mono-, and granulocytic cells per μL; protein was elevated to 2000 mg/L. There was intrathecal production of IgG, IgM, and IgA; oligoclonal bands were positive. Blood and CSF IgG-titers and CSF IgM-titers for *Borrelia burgdorferi* were increased markedly. There also was a strong increase of HCV-titers; HCV-RNA-PCR was positive with no history of hepatitis C. Cryoglobulin titers were negative.

More Case Studies in Stroke, eds. Michael G. Hennerici, Rolf Kern, Louis R. Caplan, and Kristina Szabo. Published by Cambridge University Press. © Cambridge University Press 2014.

Imaging findings

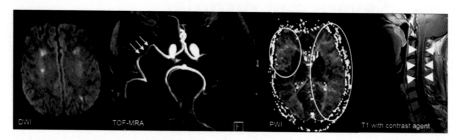

Figure 33.1. DWI image (left) shows disseminated acute ischemic lesions in both MCA territories. On MRA (middle left), there is a lack of flow in the left MCA stem and moderate narrowing of the distal right MCA (arrows). Correspondingly, there is a delay of bolus arrival in both MCA territories on perfusion MRI (middle right). Sagittal T1-weighted imaging after administration of contrast agent (right) demonstrates meningeal contrast enhancement (arrowheads).

Diagnosis

Cerebral vasculitis in Lyme neuroborreliosis.

General remarks

This is an unusual case of a young patient with slowly progressive neurological symptoms and MRI evidence of acute bihemispheric brain ischemia caused by cerebral vasculitis associated with Lyme neuroborreliosis. Lyme neuroborreliosis affects the nervous system after systemic infection with the spirochete *Borrelia burgdorferi*. The classic triad of Lyme neuroborreliosis consists of lymphocytic meningitis, cranial neuritis, and radiculoneuritis. CNS involvement is rare, but can present occasionally with encephalomyelitis or stroke. Lyme neuroborreliosis may be a differential diagnosis in patients who have unexplained cerebrovascular accidents and who live in or have travelled to areas with endemic Lyme disease. CSF analysis with evidence of lymphocytic pleocytosis and intrathecal production of *Borrelia burgdorferi*-specific antibodies is crucial for the diagnosis.

Vasculitis is probably the most overdiagnosed condition in clinical neurology. It is a very rare cause of stroke. Typically, as in this patient, the onset is over weeks to months, there are multifocal clinical and imaging abnormalities, there is a CSF pleocytosis, and the CSF protein is high.

Special remarks

Lyme neuroborreliosis should be considered a possible etiology of focal or multifocal ischemic strokes with unusual clinical and imaging presentations. Large artery vasculitis with ischemic strokes, slowly progressive symptoms, and meningeal contrast-enhancement is characteristic of neuroborreliosis-related cerebral vasculitis. The finding of positive hepatitis-C titers in this case is coincidental but likely not pathogenetically relevant.

SUGGESTED READING

Cacoub P, Saadoun D, Limal N, Léger JM, Maisonobe T. Hepatitis C virus infection and mixed cryoglobulinaemia vasculitis: a review of neurological complications. *AIDS* 2005; **19**(3): S128–34.

Halperin JJ. Stroke in Lyme disease. In Caplan LR (ed.), *Uncommon Causes of Stroke*, 2nd edn. Cambridge: Cambridge University Press, 2008.

Halperin JJ, Luft BJ, Anand AK, et al. Lyme neuroborreliosis: central nervous system manifestations. *Neurology* 1989; **39**: 753–9.

Pachner AR, Duray P, Steere AC. Cerebral nervous system manifestations of Lyme disease. *Arch Neurol* 1989; **46**: 790–5.

Schmiedel J, Gahn G, von Kummer R, Reichmann H. Cerebral vasculitis with multiple infarcts caused by Lyme disease. *Cerebrovasc Dis* 2004; **17**: 79–81.

Topakian R, Stieglbauer K, Nussbaumer K, Aichner FT. Cerebral vasculitis and stroke in Lyme neuroborreliosis. Two case reports and review of current knowledge. *Cerebrovasc Dis* 2008; **26**(5): 455–61.

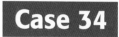
Visual field loss and memory disturbance

Marc Wolf and Rolf Kern

Clinical history

A 53-year-old woman was admitted after to a two-week history of left-sided hemicrania, scintillating scotoma in the right visual field, and poor memory. The medical history included delayed adolescence and hearing loss. The year before, at the age of 52 years, she had her first episode with headaches, seizures, and visual disturbances from which she recovered completely within three months. Her daughter was diagnosed with MELAS (mitochondrial encephalomyopathy, lactic acidosis, and stroke-like episodes) with the mitochondrial 3243 A–G mutation.

Examination

Clinical examination on admission showed difficulty giving a detailed recent history, slow responses to queries and commands, mood swings, alexia, poor hearing, and a right homonymous hemianopia.

Neurological scores: NIHSS 5, Barthel 85, mRS 3.

Special studies

Imaging findings on admission showed a large non-enhanced T2-hyperintense left temporo-occipital lesion, with cortical and hippocampal involvement and a slightly hyperintense DWI-signal with ADC reduction. The acute lesion overlapped the vascular territories of the left MCA and PCA (Figure 34.1A). Doppler-/duplex sonography was normal. An EEG showed severe temporo-occipital dysfunction with epileptiform discharges. Neuropsychological testing demonstrated aphasia and severe deficits of verbal and visual memory.

More Case Studies in Stroke, eds. Michael G. Hennerici, Rolf Kern, Louis R. Caplan, and Kristina Szabo. Published by Cambridge University Press. © Cambridge University Press 2014.

In addition to the acute lesion in the left hemisphere, a chronic right temporal lesion was detected on MRI, likely corresponding to the history of a right hemispheric stroke-like episode (Figure 34.1B).

Imaging findings

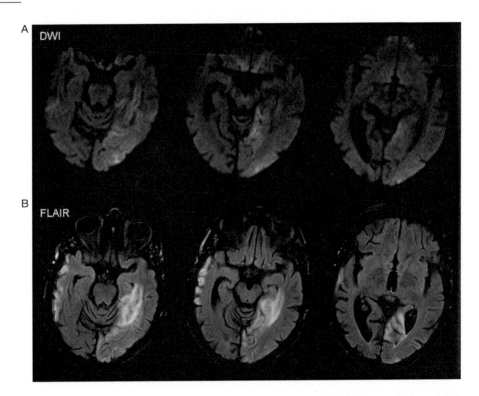

Figure 34.1. (A): DWI (upper row) shows a large lesion involving the left temporo-parieto-occipital cortex overlapping the vascular territories of the MCA and PCA. (B): On FLAIR imaging (bottom row), vasogenic edema is present in the same area, while the lesion in the right temporal cortex probably is the residuum of a first stroke-like episode in the context of MELAS syndrome.

Diagnosis

Recurrent stroke-like episode in MELAS.

General remarks

One of the typical clinical presentations of MELAS syndrome is "stroke-like episodes." Similar to the other mitochondrial cytopathies, the disease is caused by defects in the mitochondrial genome that is inherited from the female parent. The lesion pattern not matching with the distribution of vascular territories on brain imaging is one important hint to differentiate MELAS from ischemic stroke. The treatment of stroke-like episodes consists of preventing further complications, such as epileptic seizures. More specific treatment strategies have been evaluated but there is lack of clinical trials. Supplementation with L-arginine has been proposed, restoring the deficiency of L-arginine as a precursor of nitric oxide as an antioxidant. It is important to inform the patient and the family about the genetic risk of transmission, and therefore screening should be offered to potentially affected family members.

Special remarks

This patient had a first stroke-like episode some years ago with right hemispheric symptoms. FLAIR imaging showed a residual hyperintense lesion of the right temporal lobe, which probably dates from this episode. However, the patient was not diagnosed initially as having MELAS syndrome, but the diagnosis was facilitated by the positive family history and later confirmed by the finding of the same mutation. Furthermore, the additional symptoms such as delayed adolescence, hearing loss, and high serum lactate levels indicate a possible mitochondrial cytopathy.

After two weeks of antiepileptic treatment with levetiracetam, the patient was discharged with residual cognitive deficits. One year after symptom onset, MRI follow-up showed a regression of the index lesion with a rather small chronic remnant of the left-sided temporal lesion. Neuropsychological testing showed residual deficits but a considerable improvement especially of the speech.

SUGGESTED READING

Finsterer J. Management of mitochondrial stroke-like episodes. *Eur J Neurol* 2009; **16**: 1178–84.

Hirt L. MELAS and other mitochondrial disorders. In Caplan LR (ed.), *Uncommon Causes of Stroke*, 2nd edn. Cambridge: Cambridge University Press, 2008.

Ito H, Mori K, Kagami S. Neuroimaging of stroke-like episodes in MELAS. *Brain Dev* 2011; **33**: 283–8.

Koo B, Becker LE, Chuang S, et al. Mitochondrial encephalomyopathy, lactic acidosis, stroke-like episodes (MELAS): clinical, radiological, and genetic observations. *Ann Neurol* 1993; **34**: 25–32.

Matthews PM, Tampieri D, Berkovic SF, et al. Magnetic resonance imaging shows specific abnormalities in the MELAS syndrome. *Neurology* 1991; **41**: 1043–46.

Section 3

Stroke mimics

Right hemiparesis with behavioral changes

Kristina Szabo

Clinical history

A 75-year-old man was brought in by his family as an emergency after the acute onset of a slight left sensorimotor hemiparesis noticed upon awakening eight hours earlier. In retrospect, the family had noted some behavioral changes one week earlier, but could not characterize the abnormalities in detail. His previous medical history revealed long-standing hypertension, coronary heart disease, and myocardial infarction eight years earlier. The family history was negative for neuropsychiatric disorders.

Examination

He had slight, mild pyramidal distribution weakness and clumsiness, more so in the left arm than in the left leg, as well as slight hypesthesia in the left arm.
Neurological scores: NIHSS 4, Barthel 95, GCS 15.

Special studies

Initial MRI of the brain showed hyperintense lesions on DWI and a reduced ADC in the head of the caudate nucleus and the ventral part of the putamen on the right (Figure 35.1A). Duplex ultrasound of extra- and intracranial vessels showed arteriosclerotic plaques in both ICAs. In the MMSE, he achieved 29/30 points. A diagnosis of subcortical MCA and possibly ACA (parts of the head of the caudate) stroke was made and the patient was started on aspirin. After five days, he was transferred to a neurological rehabilitation unit while his clinical deficits remained unchanged.

More Case Studies in Stroke, eds. Michael G. Hennerici, Rolf Kern, Louis R. Caplan, and Kristina Szabo. Published by Cambridge University Press. © Cambridge University Press 2014.

Follow-up

One week later, the neurological rehabilitation hospital referred the patient back to our institution due to unexplained clinical worsening. On examination, his clinical condition showed a remarkable change in that he was awake but slow in cognition with a worsened MMSE score of 23/30. There was dysarthria and facial palsy on the left. In addition, he had developed a complex dystonic-hyperkinetic movement disorder, with orofacial as well as lingual hyperkinesia, and dystonic posture of the left extremities with rigidity and myoclonic jerks–characterized by both positive and negative myoclonus–mainly of his left extremities. Standing and walking was impossible without bilateral assistance.

Creutzfeldt–Jakob disease (CJD) was included in the differential diagnosis at that point and follow-up MRI as well as EEG and CSF analysis were performed, substantiating this suspicion. The EEG showed generalized slowing, while protein 14-3-3 was markedly elevated in the CSF. MRI showed the previous lesions, and in addition, slight but definite cortical hyperintensity in the right hemisphere (Figure 35.1B). The patient's condition deteriorated over the following two weeks: he was bedridden due to progression of rigidity and myoclonus of all extremities; he stopped speaking and could not swallow. Repeat MRI at three weeks showed gross progression with extension of hyperintense signal changes to cortical areas of the right frontal, temporal, parietal, and occipital lobes on DWI, as well as slightly hyperintense areas of the cortex of the left hemisphere. In addition, subtle signal increase was noted in the left caudate nucleus on DWI (Figure 35.1C). The EEG now showed periodic sharp slow wave complexes in the right frontal and temporal regions. Two months after the onset of the first clinical symptoms, the patient died. The results of the neuropathological examination confirmed the diagnosis of sporadic CJD with spongiform encephalopathy and a diffuse synaptic pattern of prion protein immunoreactivity.

Imaging findings

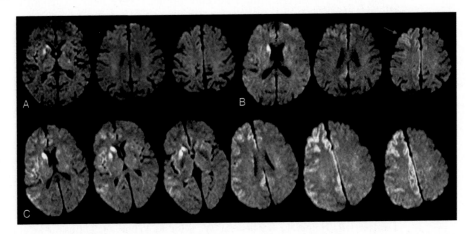

Figure 35.1. (A): initial MRI shows hyperintense signal on DWI in the head of the caudate nucleus and putamen on the right (arrow). (B): on follow-up MRI at two weeks, the hyperintense lesion in the right caudate nucleus on DWI is still seen, but in addition, faint hyperintense signal change is detected on DWI along the frontal and occipital cortex of the right hemisphere (arrows). C: MRI at week three after onset of symptoms and with clinical progression reveals increased, asymmetric hyperintense changes on DWI, now in the caudate nuclei and putamen bilaterally (R>L), and along the cortical ribbons of the frontal, parietal, temporal, and occipital lobes of the right hemisphere.

Diagnosis

Initial stroke-like presentation in a patient who had CJD.

Special remarks

Even though CJD typically presents with a rapidly progressive dementia–a syndrome atypical for acute stroke–there are a few reports describing patients with acute onset of symptoms resembling stroke. Brown et al. suggested that approximately 10% of CJD patients may show neurological symptoms at onset mimicking stroke. In a systematic review by McNaughton, 5.6% of 532 database patients with a "probable" or "definite" diagnosis of CJD fulfilled criteria for a stroke-like onset. Out of 29 of these receiving a CT scan, five were felt to have an infarct appropriate to the clinical signs.

The mechanism of reduced diffusion in CJD is unknown. Usually, reduced diffusion is detected in pathologies associated with local compromise of energy metabolism, as in acute stroke, after prolonged ictal activity, which may well be the case in CJD as mitochondrial function is impaired in the process of dying neurons. Interestingly, the reduced ADC was observed for a longer period than in acute stroke, possibly indicating continuous severe neurodegeneration in CJD. MRI-pathological correlation studies have suggested astrogliosis that is noted in T2- and DWI hyperintense lesions, and the presence of vacuoles in spongiform encephalopathy as potential causes of the low ADC values.

SUGGESTED READING

Bahn MM, Kido DK, Lin W, Pearlman AL. Brain magnetic resonance diffusion abnormalities in Creutzfeldt–Jakob disease. *Arch Neurol* 1997; **54**: 1411–15.

Brown P, Cathala F, Castaigne P, Gajdusek DC. Creutzfeldt–Jakob disease: clinical analysis of a consecutive series of 230 neuropathologically verified cases. *Ann Neurol* 1986; **20**: 597–602.

Demaerel P, Heiner L, Robberecht W, Sciot R, Wilms G. Diffusion-weighted MRI in sporadic Creutzfeldt–Jakob disease. *Neurology* 1999; **52**: 205–8.

McNaughton HK, Will RG. Creutzfeldt–Jakob disease presenting acutely as stroke; an analysis of 30 cases. *Neurol Infect Epidemiol* 1997; **2**: 19–24.

Urbach H, Klisch J, Wolf HK, et al. MRI in sporadic Creutzfeldt–Jakob disease: correlation with clinical and neuropathological data. *Neuroradiology* 1998; **40**: 65–70.

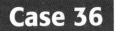

Case 36

Acute stroke symptoms in a 23-year-old man

Björn Reuter and Marc Wolf

Clinical history

A 23-year-old man presented with an acute severe right hemispheric sensorimotor syndrome (NIHSS 9) including prominent left hemineglect and anosognosia. Because he presented in the two hours after onset of the symptoms, he received systemic i.v. thrombolysis based on CT criteria. The patient showed a rapid improvement of the neurological deficits with only a mild facial asymmetry after thrombolysis (NIHSS 1). His past medical history was normal except for chronic diarrhea for unknown reasons during the last few months.

Later in the clinical course, the patient developed sudden tetraparesis and dysarthria (NIHSS 6) 24 hours after admission. Fortunately, he recovered completely within six hours and was again asymptomatic (NIHSS 0).

Special studies

Doppler-/Duplex sonography of the extra-/intracranial vessels revealed no abnormalities. TTE was normal. MRI showed a right hemispheric subcortical DWI lesion with bilateral distal occlusion of MCA branches (Figure 36.1). Additional CSF diagnostics were performed, revealing no pleocytosis. Testing for coagulopathies showed no specific alterations; however, serological screening showed a so far unknown positive HIV serology in peripheral blood as well as in the CSF. Further diagnostics revealed lymphopenia (<1000/µl, CD4 6%) and an elevated viral load (720 000/ml). Opportunistic CNS infections were excluded. In the context of the HIV infection, splenomegaly, HIV myelopathy, and HIV enteritis were diagnosed indicating a longer-lasting course of the disease.

More Case Studies in Stroke, eds. Michael G. Hennerici, Rolf Kern, Louis R. Caplan, and Kristina Szabo. Published by Cambridge University Press. © Cambridge University Press 2014.

Imaging findings

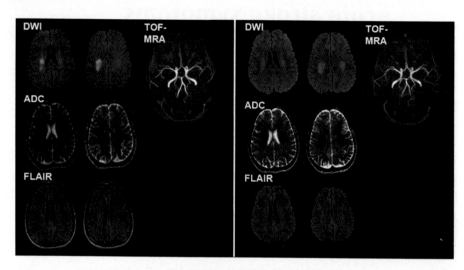

Figure 36.1. Left: MRI post-thrombolysis revealed a DWI hyperintense signal in the right periventricular white matter with a corresponding ADC reduction and additional bilateral vessel occlusion of tertiary lateral hemispheric branches of the MCA on TOF-MRA. Right: a second MRI immediately after onset of new symptoms 24 hours post-thrombolysis showed a new and almost symmetrical lesion with identical signal characteristics in the left hemisphere. TOF-MRA showed reperfusion of the formerly occluded MCA branches. Follow-up MRI examinations 12 days after admission showed gradual resolution of the subcortical edema.

Diagnosis

Stroke-like presentation of toxic leukoencephalopathy as the initial manifestation of HIV infection.

General remarks

The imaging constellation of acute DWI lesions with a hypointense correlate on ADC is typical for cytotoxic edema. In this patient, the fluctuating symptoms and imaging findings of bilateral white matter edema was most likely compatible with a toxic leukoencephalopathy.

Toxic leukoencephalopathy is rare and suspected to be caused by a partially reversible metabolic derangement and affection of myelinated structures. It usually occurs in patients with exposure to environmental toxins (for instance carbon monoxide), drugs (heroine, cocaine, methadone), or cancer chemotherapy (methotrexate, 5-FU, capecitabine). HIV infection of the CNS might have a direct toxic effect on myelin, as suspected in this case. In classical toxic leukoencephalopathy, the clinical onset of symptoms usually is not as abrupt as in our case and symptoms often include behavioral disorders or a confusional state. Therefore, detailed MRI often is performed after some delay and vascular imaging is not always included. This patient had a transient vasculopathy. The toxic process also might have had a vasoconstrictive effect, which has not been observed yet in larger series and might be important when discussing the pathophysiology of the focal edematous lesions.

Special remarks

The acute presentation of this leukoencephalopathy suggesting cerebrovascular disease is very rare. MRI was very helpful in differentiating between fluctuating symptoms or even progressive ischemic stroke versus a different pathology. The final clinical outcome of this patient was good; after resolution of the neurological symptoms, antiviral therapy was rapidly initiated and no further complications occurred.

CURRENT REVIEW

Baehring JM, Fulbright RK. Delayed leukoencephalopathy with stroke-like presentation of chemotherapy recipients. *J Neurol Neurosurg Psychiatry* 2008; **79**: 535–9.

SUGGESTED READING

McKinney AM, Kieffer SA, Paylor RT, et al. Acute toxic leukoencephalopathy: potential for reversibility clinically and on MRI with diffusion-weighted and FLAIR imaging. *Am J Roentgenol* 2009; **193**(1): 192–206.

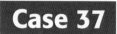

Acute onset of expressive speech disturbance

Martin Griebe

Clinical history

A 71-year-old woman was admitted to the emergency room with an acute onset of an expressive speech disturbance that had started less than two hours earlier. The relatives attending her had not observed any seizure phenomena.

They did report, however, that this right-handed patient had had a stroke one year ago with residual left-sided weakness. Her present medications did not include an anticoagulant or an antiplatelet agent, but she was taking an antiepileptic drug (gabapentin).

Examination

This alert patient presented with a severe nonfluent aphasia and a slight (presumably residual) left-sided hemiparesis.

Neurological scores: NIHSS 8, Barthel 70, GCS 13.

Special studies 1

She was considered eligible clinically for systemic thrombolytic therapy. However, MRI was preferred to CT as the primary imaging modality, because:

1. An isolated severe aphasia without right-sided hemiparesis is known to be a frequent stroke mimic.
2. The patient's history of a recent stroke, but no anticoagulant or antiplatelet medication, suggested a former hemorrhagic stroke.

The stroke-MRI did not show an acute brain infarct or hemorrhage, but did show chronic right-hemispheric parietal and occipital hemorrhagic lesions on T2*-weighted images. In addition, a linear perilesional cortical DWI hyperintensity was detected and interpreted as representing post-ictal tissue changes (Figure 37.1).

An EEG confirmed the ictal activity with right frontotemporal rhythmic discharges (Figure 37.2). Under antiepileptic therapy with levetiracetam, her

More Case Studies in Stroke, eds. Michael G. Hennerici, Rolf Kern, Louis R. Caplan, and Kristina Szabo.
Published by Cambridge University Press. © Cambridge University Press 2014.

neurological findings improved during three days and the previous clinical disability level was reached, while the EEG gradually normalized.

Imaging findings

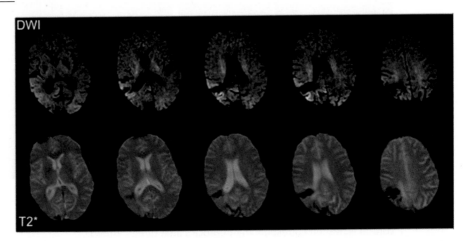

Figure 37.1. MRI shows chronic right-hemispheric parietal and occipital hemorrhagic lesions with cystic lesions and signal loss on T2*-weighted images. In addition, a perilesional cortical DWI hyperintensity is seen in the right hemisphere, involving more than one vascular territory (MCA and PCA). This was interpreted as a phenomenon induced by seizure activity.

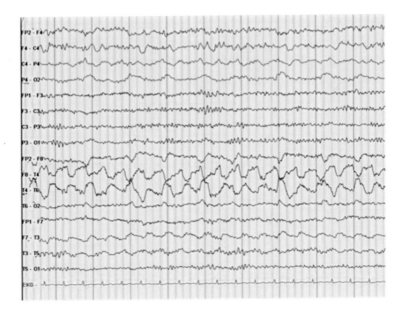

Figure 37.2. EEG shows seizure activity with right frontotemporal rhythmic discharges (F8-T4, T4-T6).

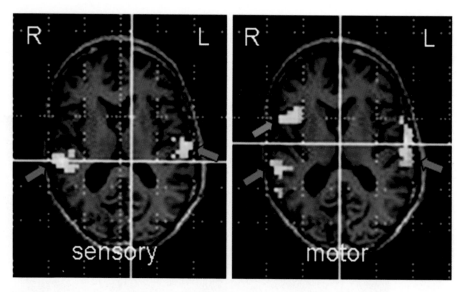

Figure 37.3. Functional MRI of language tasks shows bilateral cortical activation in the superior temporal gyri corresponding to Wernicke's area (pink arrows), and exclusively right-sided frontolateral cortical activation corresponding to Broca's area (green arrow).

Special studies 2

Neuropsychological testing identified the patient as a moderately right-handed person (Edinburgh Handedness Inventory score: +70). Using fMRI, lateralization of language representation to the right hemisphere was identified. While bilateral cortical activation in the superior temporal gyri corresponding to Wernicke's area was observed, exclusive right-sided frontolateral cortical activation corresponding to Broca's area was detected (Figure 37.3).

Diagnosis

Focal epilepsy due to chronic right-hemispheric hemorrhage with post-ictal crossed aphasia.

General remarks

Language is commonly lateralized to the left hemisphere, even in left-handed (73%) and ambidextrous individuals (85%). In a minority of right-handed persons (4%), right-hemispheric language dominance is observed. Aphasia due to lesions of the right hemisphere is termed crossed aphasia.

Special remarks

This case emphasizes the relevance of MRI as a first-line modality in acute stroke diagnosis. The patient presented with a presumed acute left-hemispheric syndrome. She was clinically eligible for systemic thrombolytic treatment and could have been falsely treated with r-tPA on the basis of standard CT imaging alone. Even though recent reports suggest that accidental thrombolysis in stroke mimics is safe, this particular patient would probably have carried a higher risk of bleeding because of her former ICH. With the increasing availability of MR scanners and a growing experience in patient handling resulting in a minimal procedural delay, MRI should be considered as the imaging technique of choice in any acute stroke patient with a non-straightforward presentation.

SUGGESTED READING

Förster A, Griebe M, Wolf ME, et al. How to identify stroke mimics in patients eligible for intravenous thrombolysis? *J Neurol* 2012; **259**: 1347–53.

Knecht S, Dräger B, Deppe M, et al. Handedness and hemispheric language dominance in healthy humans. *Brain* 2000; **123**: 2512–18.

Winkler DT, Fluri F, Fuhr P, et al. Thrombolysis in stroke mimics: frequency, clinical characteristics, and outcome. *Stroke* 2009; **40**: 1522–5.

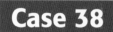

Complete loss of vision in a 44-year-old woman

Philipp Eisele

Clinical history

A 44-year-old woman was brought to the emergency department due to complete (binocular) blindness that had started approximately an hour earlier. Paramedics reported no cognitive or language disturbances; her blood pressure was very high with systolic values exceeding 230 mmHg. She also reported persistent vertigo, nausea, vomiting, and headache for the past two days.

Her medical history was notable for hypertension and type 2 insulin-dependent diabetes mellitus. She was a smoker and was obese (body mass index 33.7 kg/m^2). She had no pre-existing kidney disease and was not on immunosuppressive medication.

Examination

Neurological examination showed loss of vision in both eyes (cortical blindness) with absent optokinetic nystagmus. Her pupils reacted to light.

Neurological scores: NIHSS 3, Barthel 100, mRS 2, GCS 15.

Special studies

Routine laboratory tests were normal. As acute ischemic stroke in the visual cortex was suspected; emergency MRI was performed. MRI failed to show areas of restricted diffusion or signs of acute hemorrhage, and there were no vessel abnormalities on MRA. However, multiple symmetric T2-hyperintense lesions in both parieto-occipital regions involving the cortex and the subcortical white matter with mild contrast enhancement–interpreted as vasogenic edema–were shown. CSF showed normal cell count, although total protein was elevated (600 mg/L). An EEG initially demonstrated intermittent bilateral parieto-occipital focal slowing without epileptiform discharge (Figure 38.1).

More Case Studies in Stroke, eds. Michael G. Hennerici, Rolf Kern, Louis R. Caplan, and Kristina Szabo. Published by Cambridge University Press. © Cambridge University Press 2014.

Imaging findings

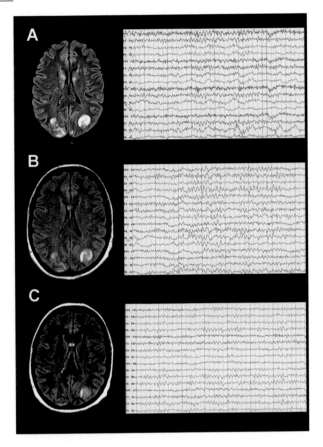

Figure 38.1. (A): T2-FLAIR MRI on admission demonstrates multiple hyperintense lesions, mainly in the parieto-occipital regions. The striate cortical zones were spared. EEG shows intermittent parieto-occipital theta-delta-range slowing bilaterally. (B): on MRI two days after admission, the lesions already are regressive, as is the parieto-occipital focal slowing. (C): five days after admission, MRI and EEG show further improvement.

Diagnosis

Posterior reversible encephalopathy syndrome (PRES) due to severe hypertension.

Follow-up

Over the course of the next seven days, under antihypertensive and antiepileptic therapy with levetiracetam, the patient improved and recovered completely; MRI and EEG normalized gradually.

General remarks

The term PRES describes a group of heterogeneous disorders with variable clinical presentation including headache, cognitive and behavioral abnormalities, seizures, and visual loss attributable to different causes such as hypertensive encephalopathy, pre-eclampsia/eclampsia, drug neurotoxicity, uremia, thrombotic thrombocytopenic purpura, and cerebral amyloid angiopathy. Even though the pathophysiology of PRES is unknown and remains controversial, several hypotheses are under debate:

1. Severe hypertension with failed autoregulation leads to injury of the capillary bed, resulting in brain edema. The findings represent a capillary leak syndrome in the brain, in the kidney, and sometimes in the retina.
2. Hypertension leads to cerebral vasoconstriction, and therefore brain edema and ischemia.

Typical findings on MRI include hyperintense signal on T2-FLAIR images, primarily in the subcortical white matter of the parieto-occipital regions but the cortex and other regions may be involved as well. Unlike a top-of-the-basilar artery embolus, which characteristically involves the striate regions, the calcarine cortex invariably is spared in patients with PRES. Mild enhancement on T1-postcontrast images has been reported but is not seen constantly.

SUGGESTED READING

Bartynski WS. Posterior reversible encephalopathy syndrome, part 1: fundamental imaging and clinical features. *Am J Neuroradiol* 2008; **29**(6): 1036–42.

Bartynski WS. Posterior reversible encephalopathy syndrome, part 2: controversies surrounding pathophysiology of vasogenic edema. *Am J Neuroradiol* 2008; **29**(6): 1043–9.

Casey SO, Sampaio RC, Michel E, Truwit CL. Posterior reversible encephalopathy syndrome: utility of fluid-attenuated inversion recovery MR imaging in the detection of cortical and subcortical lesions. *Am J Neuroradiol* 2000; **21**(7): 1199–206.

Covarrubias DJ, Luetmer PH, Campeau NG. Posterior reversible encephalopathy syndrome: prognostic utility of quantitative diffusion-weighted MR images. *Am J Neuroradiol* 2002; **23**(6): 1038–48.

Hinchey JA, Chaves CJ, Appignani B, et al. A reversible posterior leukoencephalopathy syndrome. *N Engl J Med* 1996; **334**: 494–500.

Case 39

Spells of numbness in a biochemical graduate

Louis R. Caplan

Clinical history

A 27-year-old biochemical graduate student had a series of attacks that began during the summer of 2004. In one episode, he became quite "dizzy" and felt that his eyes were being pulled to the right. He had many attacks that were characterized by spreading numbness, often beginning in his left face or left fingers that gradually spread over the face and left upper limb. The spells lasted five to 15 minutes and were often repeated several times during the day. He also had frequent headaches, sometimes developing after the spells. The attacks had been occurring for three weeks when I first was consulted. He had no past history of headaches and had had no fever or chills or systemic symptoms. His past history and family history were negative.

Examination

His blood pressure was 125/70, and pulse was regular. He had no cardiac abnormalities on examination, and his neurological examination was normal.

Special studies

A spinal tap was performed and the CSF contained 88 white blood cells, 97% lymphocytes; the protein was 67 and the sugar was normal. Culture reports were normal.

His brain imaging showed several small lesions on FLAIR MRI, one involving the right head of the caudate nucleus, and several in the white matter adjacent to the left thalamus (Figure 39.1).

I saw the patient the evening before a planned brain biopsy. I suggested that he had Bartleson syndrome and urged a course of verapamil instead of brain biopsy. He had one characteristic attack the next morning but none after

More Case Studies in Stroke, eds. Michael G. Hennerici, Rolf Kern, Louis R. Caplan, and Kristina Szabo.
Published by Cambridge University Press. © Cambridge University Press 2014.

that. When spoken to five years later, he had had no further spells and was functioning normally.

Imaging findings

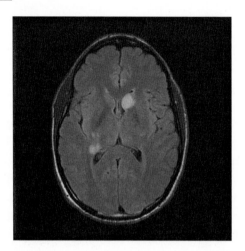

Figure 39.1. T2-weighted FLAIR MRI showed an acute hyperintense lesion in the head of the caudate nucleus on the right as well as several smaller hyperintense lesions in the white matter lateral of the left thalamus.

Diagnosis

Bartleson syndrome.

Remarks

Bartleson syndrome is an important but infrequent clinical syndrome that includes migraine-like headache and neurological signs. Bartleson syndrome (also referred to as a pseudomigraine syndrome with pleocytosis, and the syndrome of transient headache with neurological deficits and CSF lymphocytosis [HaNDL]) is characterized by attacks that closely resemble migrainous auras that occur in a flurry and are accompanied by prominent headache and CSF pleocytosis. The CSF contains a lymphocytic predominant pleocytosis (>100 cells) and an elevated protein content. Many patients have recurrent aphasia sometimes associated with visual blurring or scotomata and with right limb sensory or motor dysfunction. Right hemisphere attacks also occur. Some attacks are predominantly vestibular and cerebellar or visual. The attacks are relatively stereotyped in individual patients and usually involve either the left or right cerebral hemisphere in each attack. The attacks last between 15 minutes and an hour. Attacks may occur more than once a day and cluster during a period of three to six weeks. The condition might represent a primary migraine disorder with an inflammatory etiology but other possibilities include a viral meningovascular infection or some other undefined aseptic meningitis. The early reports preceded modern brain and vascular imaging. The last three patients that I have seen with this syndrome have had scattered brain lesions on FLAIR MRI, surprisingly not all in territories that would be predicted by the symptoms during the attacks. The clinical course of Bartleson syndrome typically is self-limited, usually lasting from four to 12 weeks. Calcium-channel blockers, especially verapamil, are effective in my experience.

SUGGESTED READING

Bartleson JD, Swanson JW, Whisnant JP. A migrainous syndrome with cerebrospinal fluid pleocytosis. *Neurology* 1981; **31**: 1257–62.

Berg MJ, Williams LS. The transient syndrome of headache with neurologic deficits and CSF lymphocytosis. *Neurology* 1995; **45**: 1648.

Fuentes B, Diez Tejedor E, Pascual J, Cova J, Querce R. Cerebral blood flow changes in pseudomigraine with pleocytosis analyzed by single photon emission computed tomography. A spreading depression mechanism. *Cephalgia* 1998; **18**: 570–3.

Fumal A, Vandenheede M, Coppola G, et al. The syndrome of transient headache with neurological deficits and CSF lymphocytosis (HaNDL): electrophysiological findings suggesting a migrainous pathophysiology. *Cephalgia* 2005; **25**(9): 754–8.

Gomez-Aranda F, Canadillas F, Marti-Masso JF, et al. Pseudomigraine with temporary neurological symptoms and lymphocytic pleocytosis. A report of 50 cases. *Brain* 1997; **120**: 1105–13.

Morrison DG, Phuah HK, Reddy AT, Dure LS, Kline LB. Ophthalmologic involvement in the syndrome of headache, neurologic deficits, and cerebrospinal fluid lymphocytosis. *Ophthalmology* 2003; **110**: 115–18.

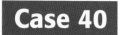

Case 40

Recurrent episodes of disturbed speech

Tilman Menzel and Rolf Kern

Clinical history

A 76-year-old woman presented with left-sided headaches, which had become more frequent and more severe during the last three months. She also reported three recent episodes of having difficulty producing speech, and each attack lasted for about 15–30 minutes. The patient had been started on oral anticoagulation medication with vitamin-K antagonists several weeks before because of recently diagnosed atrial fibrillation. She had had a brainstem stroke seven years previously with complete recovery. She was known to have hypertension and diabetes. Cancer of the colon had been curatively treated in the past.

Examination

At presentation, the neurological examination was normal.
Neurological scores: NIHSS 0, mRS 0.

Special studies

MRI showed a left temporal meningeal contrast-enhancing lesion with prominent small cortical vessels draining into the transverse venous sinus as well as surrounding edema expanding to the temporal lobe (Figure 40.1). TCCS revealed a pathological flow profile in a left-sided deep cerebral vein. On the EEG, there was left frontotemporal theta- and delta-activity without spikes or sharp waves.

Digital subtraction angiography was performed confirming a left temporal dural fistula with feeding vessels originating from the VAs and occipital and meningeal arteries, a venous ectasia and venous output stasis with concurrent thrombosis in the left sigmoid and transverse sinus (Cognard Type IV, Figure 40.2). One week later, successful embolization with ethylene–vinyl–alcohol was achieved during a second angiography, upon which MRI findings and clinical symptoms improved.

More Case Studies in Stroke, eds. Michael G. Hennerici, Rolf Kern, Louis R. Caplan, and Kristina Szabo. Published by Cambridge University Press. © Cambridge University Press 2014.

Imaging findings

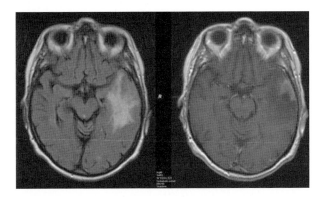

Figure 40.1. FLAIR MRI imaging (left) shows edema of the left temporal lobe. Gadolinium-enhanced T1-weighted imaging (right) demonstrates a contrast-enhancing lesion adjacent to the meninges and small prominent cortical vessels.

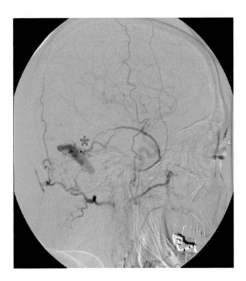

Figure 40.2. Digital subtraction angiography demonstrates the dural fistula (asterisk) with feeding vessels originating from the VAs and occipital and meningeal arteries.

Diagnosis

Cerebral dural fistula.

General remarks

Intracranial dural arteriovenous fistulas account for 10%–15% of all intracranial arteriovenous lesions. Although their symptoms and prognosis are highly variable, an association between venous drainage patterns and clinical presentation has been reported. Dural arteriovenous fistulas that drain retrogradely into cortical veins have a much higher frequency of hemorrhage or venous infarction than those with antegrade flow or drainage to larger sinuses. Venous drainage represents the basis for the Cognard classification of intracranial dural arteriovenous fistulas. Although catheter-based angiography remains the diagnostic gold standard for the imaging of dural fistulas, improvements in MRI and ultrasound technology have strengthened the diagnostic value of these noninvasive diagnostic tools.

Special remarks

Dural fistulas often are diagnosed together with a thrombosis of the neighboring venous sinuses. In some cases, dural sinus occlusions have been diagnosed before the development of fistulas so that dural sinus occlusion is a recognized cause of fistula development. In other patients, it is unclear whether a CVT was the cause for the formation of a fistula, or instead, was a consequence of the pathologically high output of a pre-existing fistula. Other putative etiological factors are previous trauma, craniotomy, and brain infarction. Ethylene–vinyl–alcohol copolymer (Onyx®) currently is favored for interventional embolization of dural arteriovenous malformations (AVMs) and fistulas with multiple feeder or output vessels. Dural fistulas tend to reoccur, in particular after only partial interventional occlusion.

SUGGESTED READING

Awad IA, Barrow DL. Conceptual overview and management strategies. In Awad IA, Barrow DL (eds.), *Dural Arteriovenous Malformations*. Park Ridge, IL: American Association of Neurological Surgeons, 1993.

Chung SJ, Kim JS, Kim JC, et al. Intracranial dural arteriovenous fistulas: analysis of 60 patients. *Cerebrovasc Dis* 2002; **13**(2): 79–88.

Cognard C, Gobin YP, Pierot L, et al. Cerebral dural arteriovenous fistulas: clinical and angiographic correlation with a revised classification of venous drainage. *Radiology* 1995; **194**(3): 671–80.

Hu YC, Newman CB, Dashti SR, Albuquerque FC, McDougall CG. Cranial dural arteriovenous fistula: transarterial Onyx embolization experience and technical nuances. *J Neurointerv Surg* 2011; **3**(1): 5–13.

Kwon BJ, Han MH, Kang HS, Chang KH. MR imaging findings of intracranial dural arteriovenous fistulas: relations with venous drainage patterns. *Am J Neuroradiol* 2005; **26**: 2500–7.

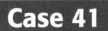

Acute aphasia and hemiparesis

Marc Wolf and Rolf Kern

Clinical history

A 70-year-old man presented with the acute onset of nearly global aphasia, somnolence, and slight right-sided hemiparesis. He could not provide any history of symptoms or medical care during the prior days and weeks. He lived alone and no other person was available or could be contacted to provide more history.

As he presented immediately after symptom onset, i.v. thrombolysis was started at 2.5 hours after exclusion of an ICH on CT.

Examination

Neurological examination revealed severe global aphasia, slight right facial weakness, and slight weakness of the right arm and leg.

Neurological scores: NIHSS 7, mRS 3.

Special studies

Unenhanced CT before i.v. thrombolysis showed chronic white matter lesions but no signs of an acute demarcated infarct or ICH. MRI after thrombolysis revealed a T2-hyperintense lesion in the left parasagittal region, with slight contrast enhancement on T1-gadolinium-based imaging (Figure 41.1). There was no ischemic lesion on DWI. Doppler-/duplex ultrasound of the extra-/ intracranial vessels showed slight atherosclerosis and stenosis of the right VA. An EEG demonstrated a left frontal theta-delta focus. Analysis of the CSF was normal. Finally, the patient was transferred to neurosurgery for brain biopsy. Pathological findings were compatible with an anaplastic astrocytoma, WHO grade III (Figure 41.2).

More Case Studies in Stroke, eds. Michael G. Hennerici, Rolf Kern, Louis R. Caplan, and Kristina Szabo. Published by Cambridge University Press. © Cambridge University Press 2014.

Imaging findings

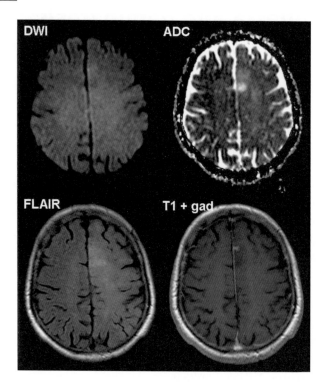

Figure 41.1. FLAIR imaging (left bottom row) shows an extensive area in the left frontal parasagittal region with slight signal hyperintensity. DWI (left upper row) is nearly normal while the ADC (right upper row) is increased at the area of the lesion. T1-weighted imaging with gadolinium (right bottom row) shows slight focal contrast enhancement near the falx.

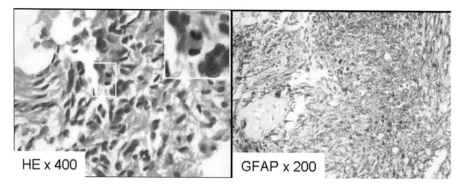

Figure 41.2. Histopathological findings show pleomorphic tumor cells on H/E staining (left) and scattered mitotic figures (left, insert). Glial fibrillary acidic protein (GFAP) expression of glial tumor cells is shown on the right. (Courtesy of Dr. W. Müller, Dept. of Neuropathology, University of Heidelberg.)

Diagnosis

Symptomatic complex-focal epileptic seizure as the first symptom of an anaplastic astrocytoma, WHO grade III.

General remarks

Brain tumor is a rare finding in patients who present with stroke mimics. Thrombolysis in stroke mimics has become an important topic with the increasing rate of thrombolysis world-wide. Because the short time period for decision making in the acute setting does not always permit an extensive imaging protocol, patients with a diagnosis other than ischemic stroke are being treated occasionally with thrombolysis. Studies have reported a rate 1%–14% of patients with stroke mimics receiving thrombolysis. However, thrombolysis in such patients seems relatively safe. Some observations showed that this subgroup of patients often present with only minor deficits such as isolated aphasia.

The key to diagnosis of cerebrovascular disease is the history of onset and risk factors. Unfortunately, the history is often cursory or neglected in the haste to obtain imaging and to deliver treatment. In this patient, unfortunately, no history was readily obtainable when he arrived in the emergency room.

Special remarks

The patient rapidly recovered and had persistent slight pronation of the right arm and dropping of the right leg. Interdisciplinary neurooncological treatment was continued, including resection of the tumor followed by radiotherapy.

SUGGESTED READING

Forster A, Griebe M, Wolf ME, et al. How to identify stroke mimics in patients eligible for intravenous thrombolysis? *J Neurol* 2012; **259**(7): 1347–53.

Tsivgoulis G, Alexandrov AV, Chang J, et al. Safety and outcome of intravenous thrombolysis in stroke mimics: a 6-year, single-care center study and a pooled analysis of reported series. *Stroke* 2011; **42**(6): 1771–4.

Zinkstok SM, Engelter ST, Gensicke H, et al. Safety of thrombolysis in stroke mimics: results from a multicenter cohort study. *Stroke* 2013; **44**(4): 1080–4.

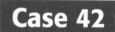

Case 42

Man with gait disturbance and urinary retention

Valentin Held

Clinical history

A 64-year-old man was referred to our hospital with progressing abnormalities of gait and sensation in his legs, and urinary dysfunction. Nine months ago, he had suddenly slumped due to a loss of strength in both legs. After about ten minutes he was able to walk again normally. A similar episode occurred on the same day, and from then on he had varying degrees of gait disturbance: sometimes he was able to walk even long distances, on other days he was not able to walk at all. About the same time, he started noticing numbness and a tingling sensation in both legs. Three months before admission he had been treated for urinary retention, which had been interpreted as due to prostatic hypertrophy, even though the prostate volume was normal.

Examination

A clinical examination on admission showed paraparesis, more pronounced proximally and on the left, with levels of strength ranging from 4/5 to 5/5. Muscle tone was slightly elevated and tendon reflexes were hyperactive in the legs; Babinski's sign was negative. Sensation was reduced caudal to the fifth thoracic segment.

Special studies

Motor EPs revealed a mild lesion of the pyramidal tract; sensory EPs showed an afferent conduction defect from the left leg. Nerve conduction studies were consistent with a slight right L5 radiculopathy. Lumbar puncture was normal except for slightly elevated total protein.

On T2-weighted MRI of the spine, hyperintensity of the spinal cord from T3 downward was visible, as well as pronounced vessels on the suface of the

More Case Studies in Stroke, eds. Michael G. Hennerici, Rolf Kern, Louis R. Caplan, and Kristina Szabo. Published by Cambridge University Press. © Cambridge University Press 2014.

spinal cord in the lower cervical and upper thoracic segments. Contrast-enhanced spinal MRA revealed early venous contrast; an evident feeder could not be identified. Only slight degenerative changes of the cervical and lumbar spine were observed. Subsequent digital subtraction angiography revealed a single feeder on the right side at T5, branching off a radicular artery and draining into an arteriovenous fistula. Embolization of the feeder safely was not possible, therefore a single platinum coil was placed as an aid to the neurosurgeon (Figure 42.1).

Imaging findings

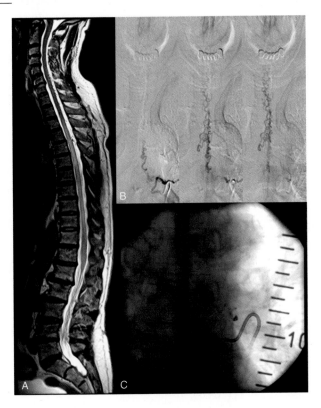

Figure 42.1. (A): T2-weighted spinal MRI shows dilated vessels intradurally. The spinal cord is hyperintense from the upper thoracic segments down to the conus. (B): the feeder at level T5 is shown draining cranially in digital subtraction angiography. (C): a coil is placed to aid the neurosurgeon.

Diagnosis

Spinal arteriovenous malformation.

General remarks

Spinal arterial malformations lie intradurally but extramedullary. They are fed by a radiculomeningeal artery and drain to a radicular vein. This leads to increased pressure in the venous system, and thus reduced perfusion of the tissue and edema, which may be widespread. While initially reversible, congestive ischemia may evolve in later stages of the disease. Spinal AVMs may be found anywhere along the spine but occur most commonly in the lower thoracic or upper lumbar segments. Furthermore, symptoms may vary according to lateralization and the predominant involvement of spinal tracts, neurons, or radices. Spinal AVMs are thought to be acquired, although the mechanisms involved remain unclear. Paraparesis (either flaccid or spastic), sensory symptoms, and bladder and bowel dysfunction are the most common symptoms of spinal AVMs. Lower back pain is common, but nonspecific and very rarely due to a hemorrhage. Onset may be insidious or sudden and symptom severity often fluctuates. Some patients have spinal TIAs. When symptom onset is sudden, and especially when symptoms are asymmetrical, spinal AVMs may mimic acute stroke.

Special remarks

Treatment is either endovascular or surgical. While the former is less invasive, the latter may occlude the shunt more effectively. After occlusion most patients recover, at least partially, with motor and sensory symptoms usually improving more completely than bladder and bowel functions. This course was also present in the patient reported here.

SUGGESTED READING

Antonietti L, Sheth SA, Halbach VV, et al. Long-term outcome in the repair of spinal cord perimedullary arteriovenous fistulas. *Am J Neuroradiol* 2010; **31**(10): 1824–30.

Ferrell AS, Tubbs RS, Acakpo-Satchivi L, Deveikis JP, Harrigan MR. Legacy and current understanding of the often-misunderstood Foix–Alajouanine syndrome. Historical vignette. *J Neurosurg* 2009; **111**: 902–6.

Jellema K, Canta LR, Tijssen CC, et al. Spinal dural arteriovenous fistulas: clinical features in 80 patients. *J Neurol Neurosurg Psychiatry* 2003; **74**: 1438–40.

Krings T, Geibprasert S. Spinal dural arteriovenous fistulas. *Am J Neuroradiol* 2009; **30**(4): 639–48.

Index